REGIONAL ARTHROSCOPY

Edited by **Vaibhav Bagaria**

Regional Arthroscopy
http://dx.doi.org/10.5772/45960
Edited by Vaibhav Bagaria

Contributors

Jami Ilyas, Jeremy Rushbrook, Panos Souroullas, Neil Pennington, Edvitar Leibur, Stefan Cristea, Fl. Groseanu, Andrei Prundeanu, D. Gartonea, Andrei Papp, Dorel Bratu, Mihai Gavrila, Juan Ponte, Ricardo Cuellar, Yuelin Hu, Chen Jiao, Qinwei Guo, Vaibhav Bagaria, Vikram Sapre

Published by InTech

Janeza Trdine 9, 51000 Rijeka, Croatia

Publishing Process Manager Danijela Duric
Technical Editor InTech DTP team
Cover InTech Design team

Additional hard copies can be obtained from orders@intechopen.com

Regional Arthroscopy , Edited by Vaibhav Bagaria
p. cm.
ISBN 978-953-51-1044-6

For EU product safety concerns:
IN TECH d.o.o., Prolaz Marije Krucifikse Kozulić 3, 51000 Rijeka, Croatia,
info@intechopen.com or visit our website at intechopen.com.

Meet the editor

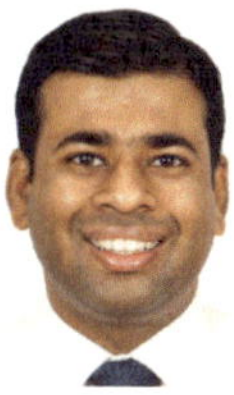

Dr Vaibhav Bagaria is currently working as a senior consultant joint replacement and sports injury surgeon at the Care hospital, Nagpur. He did his post graduation (MS) in Orthopaedics from the prestigious KEM Hospital, Mumbai after completing his MBBS from Govt. Medical College (GMC), Nagpur during which he received three gold medals. He then worked at Medical College of Wisconsin, Milwaukee, USA for a year during which he also received two international awards and diploma from SICOT, Belgium. He then undertook fellowship in advanced joint replacement and adult reconstruction in Germany and later at Perth, Adelaide & Melbourne in Australia. He is the first Indian to top the international Diploma SICOT exam.
He has received many national and international awards. His name has been included in the current years Marquis Who's who for achievements in his field. He was chosen to solely represent the medical community in the Beijing Olympic torch relay held in India in 2008. He is also the recipient of the prestigious Korean award and Lester Lowe award at World Orthopedic congress held at Istanbul 2005. He is serving on the editorial board of many journals and has also authored many papers in national and international journals and has written many books and book chapters.

Contents

Preface

Machiavelli once stated, "and one ought to consider that there is nothing more difficult to pull off, more chancy to succeed in, or more dangerous to manage, than the introduction of a new order of things." It was similar experience that the founding fathers of arthrosocopy faced when they started this unique way of treating the musculoskeletal conditions.

Arthroscopy has now become the most commonly performed musculoskeletal procedure. Arthroscopy has had several beneficial effects especially in terms of reduction of morbidity and reducing and in many cases eliminating the need for hospitalization. It all began with the knee surgeries and even today the most common arthroscopic procedures are performed in knee and yet arthroscopic surgeries performed for other regions right from temperomandibular joint down to the subtalar joint have replicated the success shown in knee surgeries. They are gradually becoming popular and this book intend to describe the tips and tricks employed by the experts in their respective field for benefit of the residents and fellows.

This book has brought the experts in the field of the arthroscopy who have written the chapters concerning various regions vizTemporomandibular joint, Shoulder, Wrist, Lumbar Spine, Knee, Ankle, and the Subtalar Joint. The focus has been on delivering key surgical points that will help ensure that learning is seamless. There is vast literature on knee arthroscopy but the information on arthroscopic procedures of other region and I hope that this book will in the lacunae.

The book of this magnitude requires a great deal of perseverance, attention to details and close coordination. Towards this end, the team at Intech had been fabulous at every step. So has been my beautiful wife Shalini and my son Shaurya who many times missed his football lessons on account of my being busy with the book. This book is dedicated to my patients, students and my parents who have taught me lessons in orthopedics and life selflessly. I hope that the book will meet their expectation and will especiallyencourage students to thoughtfully experiment and cross borders in the filed of 'Minimally Invasive keyhole procedures'.

Dr Vaibhav Bagaria
MBBS, MS, FCPS, Dip SICOT (Belgium),
Fellow Orthopedic Surgeon: USA, Australia, Germany
Senior Consultant Orthopedic & Joint Replacement Surgeon

Chapter 1

Ankle Arthroscopy

Jami Ilyas

Additional information is available at the end of the chapter

http://dx.doi.org/10.5772/54013

1. Introduction

Arthroscopy is a valuable skill for the foot and ankle surgeon and is used not only to evaluate and treat intra-articular abnormalities but also for endoscopic and tendoscopic procedures. Burman [1] was the first to attempt arthroscopy of the ankle joint in 1931 and surmised that it was not a suitable joint for arthroscopy because of its narrow intra-articular space. With the development of smaller-diameter arthroscopes and improvements in joint distraction techniques, there was a renewed interest in ankle arthroscopy. Watanabe [2] was the first to present a series of 28 ankle arthroscopies in 1972.

Arthroscopic surgery of the ankle allows the direct visualization of all intra-articular structures of the ankle without an arthrotomy or malleolar osteotomy. Technological advances and a thorough understanding of anatomy have resulted in an improved ability to perform diagnostic and operative arthroscopy of the ankle. The decreased morbidity and faster recovery times make it an appealing technique compared with open arthrotomy.

2. Indications and contraindications of ankle arthroscopy

For the purpose of simplification, relative indications for ankle arthroscopy can be divided into 3 distinct surgical categories based on the desired final outcome for the procedure:

1. Arthroscopic ankle survey
2. Arthroscopic reparative ankle surgery
3. Arthroscopic ablative ankle surgery

2.1. Arthroscopic ankle survey

Arthroscopic survey should be considered when preoperative assessment of the ankle joint does not yield a confirmative diagnosis via clinical, physical, or diagnostic testing. Arthroscopic survey in the ankle joint may also be desired as a precursor to anticipated reparative arthroscopic procedures as well.

Indications for an ankle arthroscopic survey include lavage for septic joint with survey, syndesmotic analysis, preemptive assessment of joint before an intended open repair, assessment of poorly placed internal or external fixation hardware & arthroscopic biopsy. With respect to arthroscopic survey, the scope of the procedure is relatively narrow, as one would expect with any operative survey. Surveys may be performed after an examination under anaesthesia with mortise and Broden's views of the ankle under image intensification before a formal repair of the lateral ligament & retinacular structures or "Brostrom" (modified/ true) repair for ankle joint instability.

An arthroscopic survey may also be beneficial as a diagnostic tool when infection is suspected. The success of this approach may be directly related to the physiologic lavage and reduction of a pathologic microorganism count more so than the topical introduction of antibiotic-rich saline. Often, an unsuspected chondral fracture or soft-tissue lesion not detected on radiographic, clinical, or laboratory evaluation or on bone scanning or magnetic resonance (MRI) imaging can become obvious on arthroscopic examination [3].

2.2. Arthroscopic reparative ankle surgery

Reparative arthroscopy may be indicated when preoperative assessment examinations are relatively conclusive for an underlying pathology via clinical, physical, or diagnostic findings. Simply put, this is a surgical "search and remove/repair" approach to ankle arthroscopy. Reparative indications include synovectomy, ligament repair, osteochondral defect repair, capsular thermo-cautery, intra-articular fracture reduction, arthrofibrosis, impingement syndromes (either soft tissue or osseous), and os trigonum resection.

2.3. Arthroscopic ablative ankle surgery

Another parameter in the surgical decision-making process as to whether an open repair versus an arthroscopic procedure is better indicated can be made on realization of the constraints of an arthroscopic approach to the ankle joint. Studies have shown that patients with bony or soft tissue impingements tend to do better with smaller focal impingements and a lack of significant osteoarthritis. This consideration is an important one if solely for the purpose of open treatment consent and appropriate instrumentation being available at time of surgery. Arthroscopy can also be used in ankle-stabilization procedures [7] and arthrodesis [11, 12] as well as for irrigation and debridement of septic arthritis [13].

Relative contraindications for arthroscopy of the ankle include moderate degenerative joint disease with a restricted range of motion, a markedly reduced joint space, severe edema, reflex sympathetic dystrophy, and a tenuous vascular status. More absolute contraindications include localized soft-tissue infection and severe degenerative joint disease [9].

http://dx.doi.org/10.5772/54013

Soft tissue Lesions	Bony Indications
• Synovitis	• Osteochondral lesions
• Anterior soft tissue impingement	• Loose bodies
• Posterior soft tissue impingement	• Osteophytes
• Syndesmotic impingement	• Traumatic and degenerative osteoarthritis
• Lateral ankle instability	• Ankle fusion
	• Acute ankle fractures

Table 1. Indications for Ankle Arthroscopy

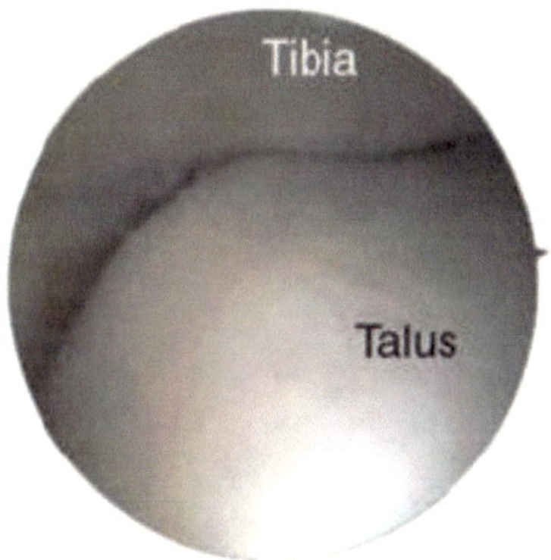

Figure 1. Normal ankle joint,

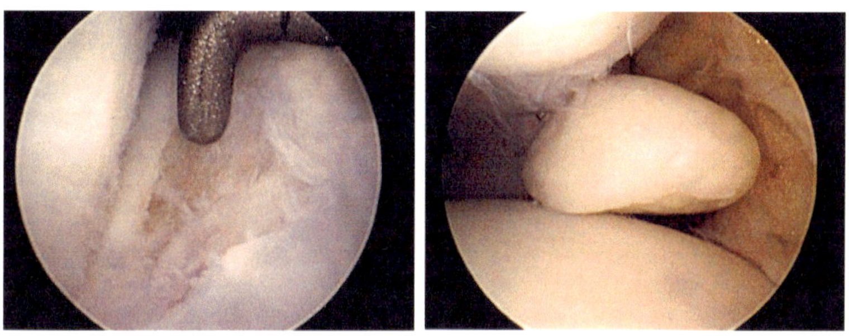

Figure 2. a) Osteoarthritis and **b)** Loose body

3. Synovitis

The synovial lining of the ankle joint may become inflamed and hypertrophied secondary to various inflammatory arthritis, infection, and degenerative or neuropathic changes. Trauma and overuse can cause generalized inflammation of the joint synovium, resulting in pain and swelling.

Diagnosis may be made clinically on the basis of diffuse ankle pain and swelling with painful range of motion. Septic arthritis, gout, and other systemic arthritis must first be ruled out with aspiration. Localized synovitis of the medial or lateral talo-malleolar joint can develop after trauma (Figure 3). Localized tenderness with minimal swelling and full range of motion is usually seen on physical examination. The diagnostic workup is usually negative, although there may be some signal alteration on MR imaging.

Initial treatment should consist of limited weight bearing, anti-inflammatory medication, and physical therapy. Intra-articular injections of corticosteroids may be used. Failure of conservative treatment of at least 3 months duration is the indication for arthroscopic partial synovectomy and lysis of adhesions, which can provide dramatic relief of pain. Treatment of infected ankle joints by arthroscopic irrigation and debridement has been described [28]. The less invasive nature of the procedure is appealing. However, there are no prospective studies comparing open and arthroscopic debridement of infected ankle joints, and the latter should therefore be considered an investigational technique.

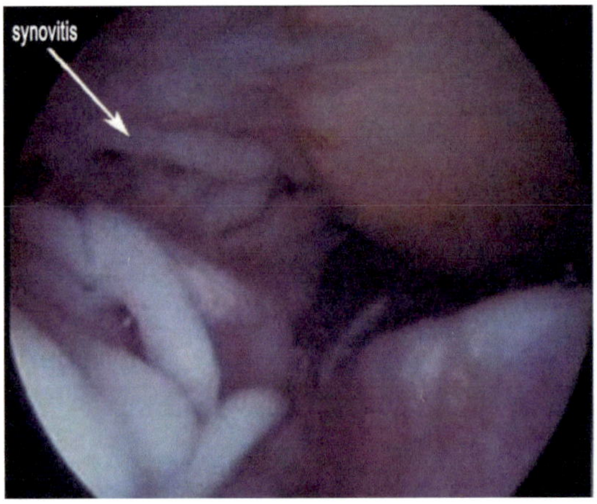

Figure 3. Synovitis and arthrofibrosis in ankle joint

4. Soft tissue impingement

4.1. Anterior soft tissue Impingement

The cause of chronic lateral ankle pain is often elusive, particularly in patients whose ankles are stable on physical examination and stress radiography. Anterior soft-tissue impingement, or anterolateral impingement of the ankle, is believed to be caused by one or more inversion injuries to the ankle joint [4]. The pain is usually anterolateral and persists despite adequate rest, healing, and rehabilitation.

http://dx.doi.org/10.5772/54013

Physical examination must distinguish pain in the lateral gutter of the ankle joint from pain in the area of the sinus tarsi. If there is tenderness in both areas, an anesthetic agent should be injected into the sinus tarsi; if this relieves the symptoms, the diagnosis of anterolateral impingement should not be made. The two may coexist, or subtalar dysfunction may be the underlying problem. The differential diagnosis includes ankle and subtalar instability, osteochondral lesions of the talus, calcific ossicle beneath the malleolus, peroneal subluxation or tear, tarsal coalition, and degeneative joint disease [4].

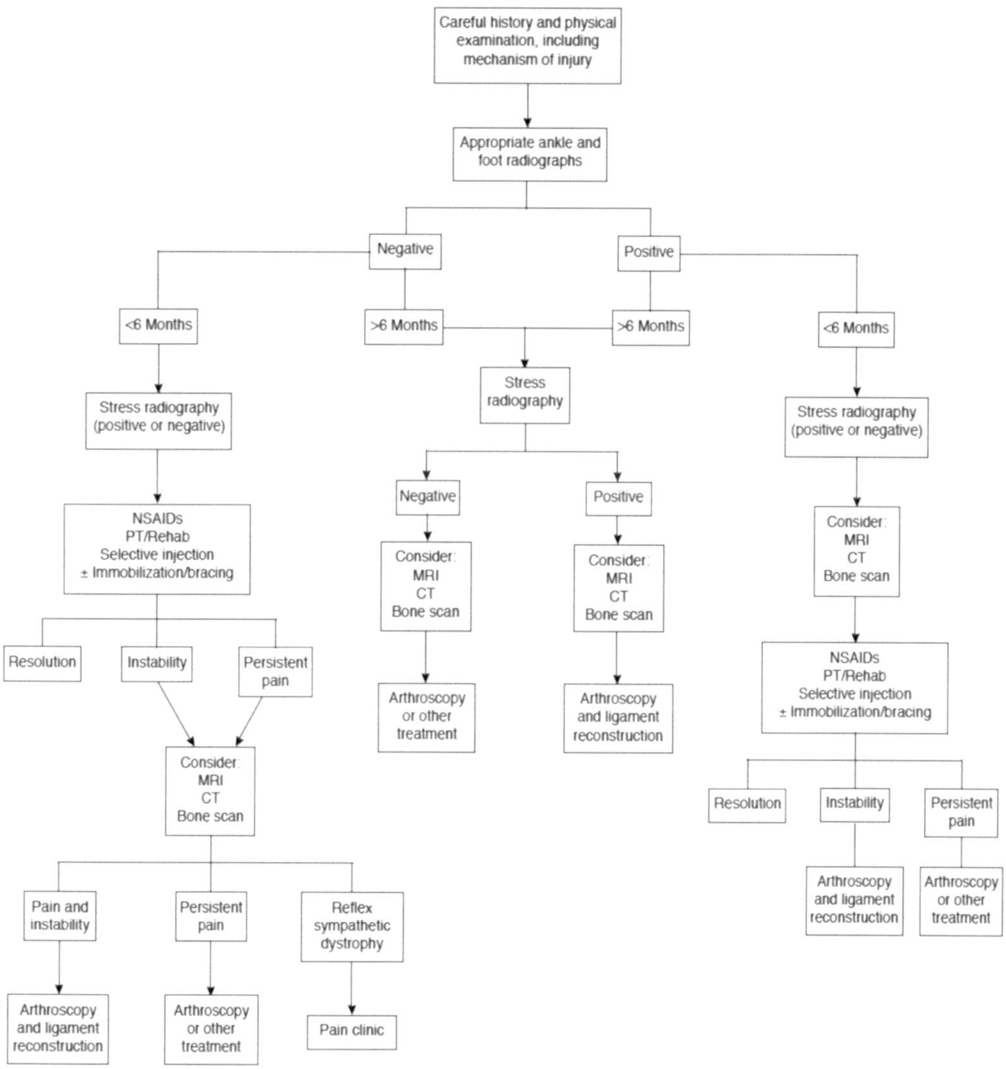

Figure 4. Algorithm for management of chronic ankle pain (Reference: Stetson & Ferkel, Ankle Arthroscopy: Indications & Results.J Am Acad Orthop Surg 1996 [30])

Anterolateral impingement most commonly occurs in the superior portion of the anterior talofibular ligament, but it can also be localized to the distal portion of the anteroinferior tibiofibular ligament (AITFL). Ferkel et al have stated that anterolateral synovial tissue and redundant ligamentous tissue may cause joint irritation and pain and may be secondary to an isolated tear of the anterior talofibular ligament and/or syndesmosis. Adjacent talar or fibular chondromalacia and inflammatory synovitis may be seen in association with these lesions. In some cases, soft-tissue impingement may also be seen along the entire anterolateral gutter and into the syndesmosis. Plain-radiographic studies can appear normal in patients with anterolateral impingement of the ankle. MR imaging can be more useful; it has revealed thickening of the synovium in the anterolateral gutter in almost 40% of patients. However, MR imaging may also give false-negative results. Smaller coils and different planes of imaging are needed to demonstrate impingement abnormalities more clearly. Meyer et al [29] demonstrated the value of high-resolution CT in the diagnosis of chronically painful ankle sprains. They found avulsed intra- articular or juxta-articular fragments of traumatic origin that were not readily apparent on standard radiographs of 13 patients.

A complete course of at least 4 to 6 months of conservative treatment for anterolateral impingement should be completed before arthroscopic debridement is considered. Careful arthroscopic debridement of the inflamed synovium and inflamed capsular or ligamentous tissue may be accomplished with either basket forceps or a power shaver. The cutting blade of the shaver must always be directly viewed, and the mouth of the shaver should never be turned dorsally and anteriorly, where neurovascular structures lie. Care must be taken to preserve the functional remnants of the anterior talofibular ligament. The rehabilitation program should be delayed for 2 to 3 weeks after surgery to avoid inflammation of the joint.

Histologically, moderate synovial hyperplasia with sub-synovial capsular proliferation is seen, which is indicative of chronic synovitis. Hyaline cartilage degenerative changes and fibrosis are also noted in many patients. Good to excellent results have been found in 75% to 90% of patients in whom conservative treatment was a failure [4, 5]. An algorithm has been developed to assist in appropriate treatment for a patient with chronic ankle pain.

4.2. Posterior soft-tissue impingement

Posterolateral impingement may occur in combination with anterolateral impingement. Radiography and MR imaging are often unrevealing. Generalized synovitis, fibrosis, and capsulitis are noted in the posterolateral corner of the ankle joint near the posteroinferior tibiofibular ligament (PITFL). Posterior impingement may occur with hypertrophy or tearing of the PITFL, transverse tibiofibular ligament, tibial slip, or pathologic labrum of the posterior ankle joint. There is a higher incidence of impingement type problems when both the PITFL and the transverse tibiofibular ligament are injured.

The tibial slip, which runs from the posterior talofibular ligament to the transverse ligament, may be a source of posterior soft-tissue impingement. This ligament can undergo hypertrophy and fibrosis after ankle trauma. A torn labrum can cause pathologic posterior impingement in much the same way that the superior labrum of the shoulder can cause impingement.

Pathology	Example
Trigonal process	• Fracture (acute or chronic)
	• Synchondrosis injury
	• True compression
FHL dysfunction	• Tenosynovitis
Tibiotalar	• Posterior capsuloligamentous injury
	• Osteochondritis
	• Fracture
Subtalar pathology	• Osteochondritis
	• Arthritis
Other	• Calcified inflammatory tissue
	• Prominent calcaneus posterior process
Combined	• FHL tenosynovitis and synchondrosis injury

Table 2. Etiological Classification of PAIS

Arthroscopic evaluation of all posterolateral lesions is facilitated by use of a distraction device. Views from both the anterior and posterolateral portals should also be obtained. Posterior impingement syndrome can effectively treated by means of a two-portal hindfoot approach with the patient in the prone position. This approach offers excellent access to the posterior ankle compartment, the subtalar joint, and extra-articular structures.

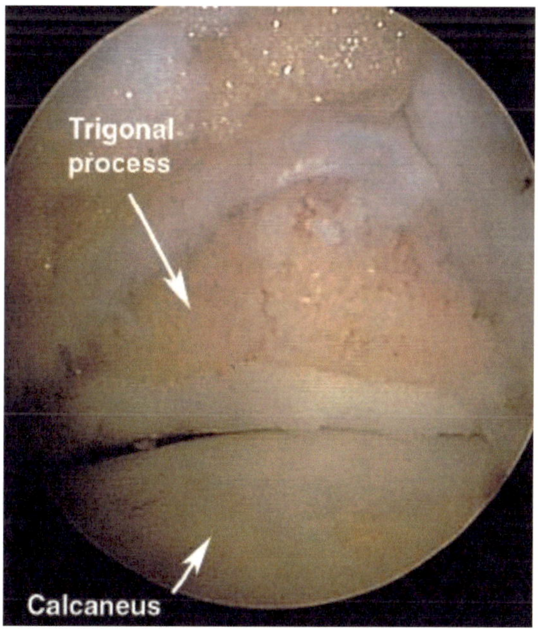

Figure 5. Posterior ankle endoscopy. Posterior ankle view after trigonal process resection.

5. Syndesmotic injury

Close [22] and Inman [23] have shown that normal movement of the ankle depends on a precise relationship determined by the syndesmosis. The talus normally articulates with the ankle mortise throughout the range of movement and the intermalleolar distance increases by approximately 1.5 mm as the ankle goes from plantar flexion to dorsiflexion. If the syndesmosis is disrupted, there may be widening of the tibiofibular joint and lateral shift of the talus. Ogilvie-Harris [11] reported that division of each ligament resulted in progressive weakening of the joint between the tibia and fibula, and Ramsey and Hamilton [24] reported that when the talus moved laterally by 1 mm the contact area of the tibiotalar articulation was decreased by 42%. Furthermore, Burns et al showed that a complete disruption of the syndesmosis combined with a tear of the deltoid ligament caused a decrease of 40% in the tibiotalar contact area and an increase of 36% in the tibiotalar contact pressure. Thus, as large changes may occur after minor ligamentous disruptions, correct diagnosis is essential for the treatment of the injured ankle (Figure 6).

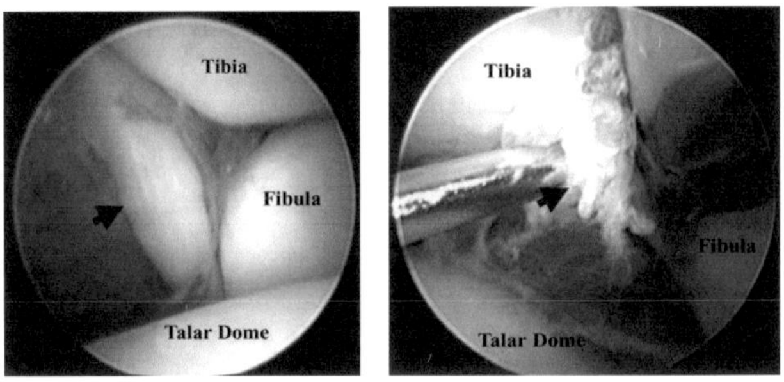

Figure 6. The AITFL. The left figure shows a normal (arrow) and the right a disrupted (arrow) ligament. It is torn in the mid-substance. The arthroscope was inserted through the anteromedial portal

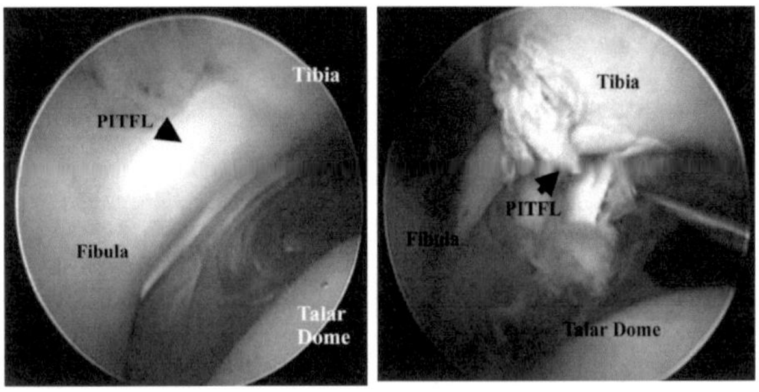

Figure 7. The PITFL. The left figure shows a normal (arrow) and the right a disrupted (arrow) ligament. It is torn from its tibial attachment. The arthroscope was inserted through the anterolateral portal

Syndesmotic injury, however, may be difficult to diagnose by radiological examination when the tears are incomplete or if there is no opening of the distal tibiofibular joint. Litera-

http://dx.doi.org/10.5772/54013

ture shows no definitive diagnostic criteria for MRI to establish incomplete syndesmotic injury, though it is very sensitive (96%) for complete tears.

The anterior tibiofibular ligament is best viewed from the anteromedial and the posterior tibiofibular ligament from the anterolateral portal. A stress test of the distal tibiofibular joint can be performed by moving the ankle from internal rotation to external rotation under arthroscopy. It has been reported that the maximum opening of the distal tibiofibular joint is approximately 1.5 mm in the normal ankle therefore, an opening of 2 mm is considered as instability (Figure 8). The diagnostic criteria for a torn ligament is abnormal course or discontinuity of the ligament, a decrease in its tension, an avulsion at its attachment to the fibula and tibia, and a positive arthroscopic stress test. By direct visualisation of the ligament and probing, arthroscopy of the ankle is an indispensable tool for the accurate diagnosis of a tear of the tibiofibular syndesmosis.

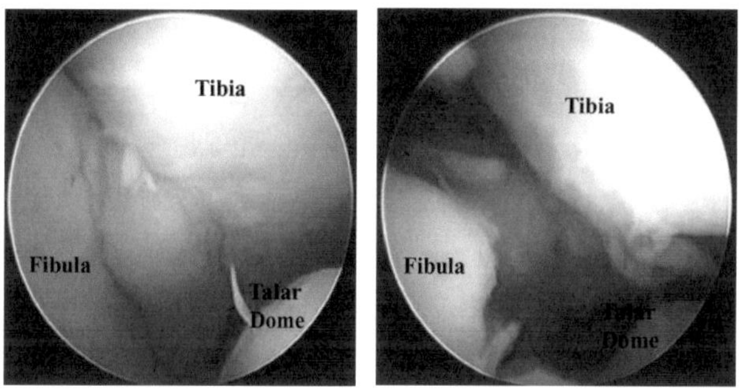

Figure 8. Stress test showing anterior tibiofibular space a) in internal and b) external rotation. The anterior tibiofibular space is widened >2 mm from internal to external rotation.

6. Lateral ankle instability

Joint instability usually coexists with intra-articular symptoms in patients with chronic ankle instability (CAI). Mechanical joint instability results from relaxed or deficient ligaments (ATFL and CFL), and functional instability is caused by weakened proprioception and other neuromuscular abnormalities. The intra-articular symptoms may be due to primary or secondary intra-articular lesions. The basic Broström procedure, which reconstructs lateral ankle stability by overlapping suture of the ATFL, is commonly used for the treatment of CAI. The modified Broström procedure, however, is used to reconstruct joint stability:

1. Tightening of the ATFL and/or CFL
2. Ligament augmentation by use of the extensor retinaculum
3. Use of a piece of periosteum to overlay the remnant of the ligament if the ligament intensity was still inadequate, despite above measures.

These measures improve the ankle stability by maximizing the ligament intensity and tension. Although the modified Broström procedure can improve ankle stability, it does not resolve the intraarticular lesions associated with CAI. The presence of accompanying intra-articular lesions might, therefore, result in a poor outcome [25]. DiGiovanni et al [27] suggested that opening inspection and management of the intra-articular lesions, in addition to the ligament reconstruction, improved the surgical outcome. However, open inspection increases surgical trauma and has been reported to only allow exploration of 20% of intra-articular lesions, as compared with those found by arthroscopy [26]. The modified Broström procedure combined with ankle arthroscopy produced significantly better surgical outcomes in patients with CAI accompanied by intra-articular symptoms.

7. Osteochondral lesion

Conservative treatment is usually advocated for grade A and grade B lesions (Ferkel- Cheng Arthroscopic Grading System: Table 3). This should include 6 to 12 weeks of casting, with the length determined by the size of the lesion. There is no good evidence that non-weight bearing in a cast is any better than weight bearing; therefore, it is not advocated. If the patient is still symptomatic after a conservative program, surgical treatment is suggested.

Grade	Arthroscopic Appearance
A	Smooth and intact, but soft or ballottable
B	Rough surface
C	Fibrillations or fissures
D	Flap present or bone exposed
E	Loose, non-displaced fragment
F	Displaced fragment

Table 3. Ferkel-Cheng Arthroscopic Grading System for Osteochondral Lesions of the Talus

Surgery is advocated for all symptomatic stage III and IV lesions, except in children whose growth plates have not closed at the distal tibial and fibular epiphyses. In these cases, initial conservative treatment with casting is recommended before surgical intervention.

Arthroscopic treatment is based on the location and extent of osteochondral injury and on whether the lesion is acute or chronic (Figure 9). For acute lesions, CT or MR imaging may be utilized to further visualize the appearance and radiologic stage. If an acute lesion is displaced, arthroscopy should be done immediately. If the lesion is primarily chondral, excision is recommended, with subsequent debridement and drilling of the base to promote formation of a fibrocartilaginous surface. Generally, drilling techniques are recommended for lesions greater than 1 cm, whereas abrasion may be adequate for smaller lesions. If the

http://dx.doi.org/10.5772/54013

chondral fragment has enough underlying bone, the piece should be reattached with absorbable pins, Kirschner wires, or Herbert screws by means of arthroscopy.

Chronic osteochondral lesions should be carefully assessed for size, location, and stability. If the lesion is not loose, transmalleolar or transtalar drilling can be accomplished. If the lesion is loose and the articular cartilage is healthy, fixation can be accomplished with absorbable pins, Kirschner wires, or screws. Most commonly, chronic lesions are loose, nonviable, and occasionally displaced and must be excised. After excision, curettage and abrasion or drilling is done.

For medial osteochondral lesions, a small-joint drill guide is inserted through the anteromedial portal, and a small puncture is made over the medial malleolus. A 0.062-mm Kirschner wire is then used to perform transmalleolar drilling into the medial aspect of the talar dome at approximately 3- to 5-mm intervals to a depth of approximately 10 mm. After drilling or abrasion, the tourniquet is released, so that the bleeding talar bed can be viewed. Postoperatively, a bulky compression dressing is applied, with a posterior splint holding the ankle in neutral position. Early range-of-motion exercises are begun at approximately 1 week, but weight bearing is delayed 4 to 8 weeks, depending on the size of the lesion

Ferkel et al. showed in his study with an average follow-up of 40 months, and found that good to excellent results were achieved in 84%. Results are worse when preexisting arthritis is present. When the results of open treatment are compared with those of arthroscopic treatment, the outcomes yielded with the latter are equally good or better.

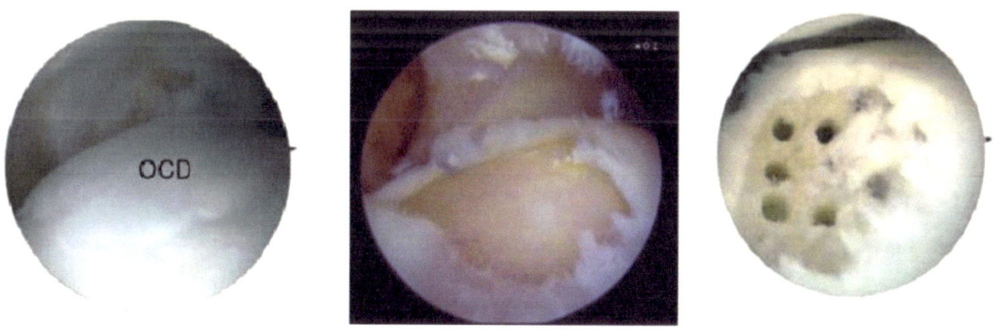

Figure 9. Osteeaoarthritis (OCD): Talus before and after drilling

8. Ankle fusion

The principles of arthroscopic ankle arthrodesis are similar to those of open arthrodesis. This includes debridement of all hyaline cartilage and underlying avascular subchondral bone from the talus, tibial plafond, and medial and lateral gutters; reduction in an appropriate position for fusion; and rigid internal fixation. During debridement, care should be taken to maintain the normal bone contour of the talar dome and the tibial plafond (i.e., talar convexity and tibial concavity).

It is critical not to remove too much bone and not to square off the tibiotalar surfaces, which could lead to a varus/valgus deformity and delayed union. The use of hand-held ring-and-cup curettes, shavers, and burrs is essential. In addition, the debridement process involves removal of the usually large anterior "lip osteophyte" so that it will not block reduction of the talar dome convexity into the concavity of the tibial plafond. Occasionally, the anterior capsule adheres to the osteophyte, and great caution must be exercised in peeling the capsule off the anterior distal tibia, so as not to injure the neurovascular structures.Fixation is usually accomplished with insertion of percutaneous transarticular 6.5- or 7.0-mm cannulated screws through the medial and lateral malleoli or two screws through the medial malleolus. Occasionally, three screws are required to secure fixation, especially if there is osteoporotic bone. External compression frames can also be used. Rarely is an anterior or posterior screw needed (Figure 10).

The disadvantages of arthroscopic arthrodesis include a difficult learning curve for the surgeon, the expense of arthroscopic equipment, and the inability to correct significant varus, valgus, and rotational problems. Another potential disadvantage of the arthroscopic technique is that it makes posterior displacement of the talus difficult.

There is a decreased time to union. This is probably because periosteal stripping was not necessary and therefore the local circulation is intact. Following arthroscopic fusion, the mean time for union may be as short as approximately 8 weeks. Some studies have found that the procedure can be done as an outpatient/overnight stay. Compared with open fusion, arthroscopic ankle arthrodesis appears to offer similar or better overall results in selected patients. The technique is particularly appealing in elderly patients and in patients with rheumatoid arthritis who are unable to tolerate prolonged non-weight-bearing postoperatively.

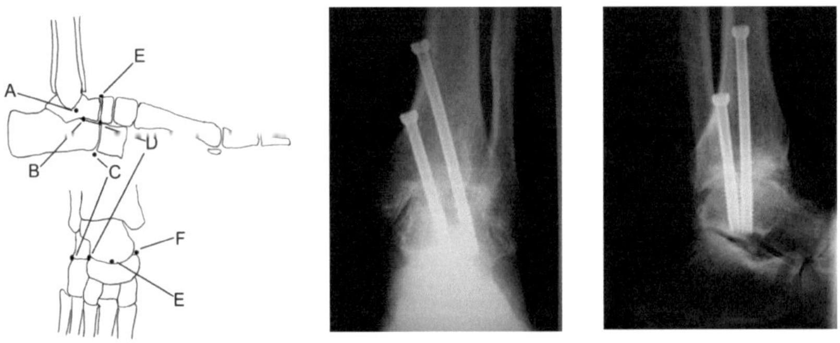

Figure 10. Arthroscopic triple arthrodesis: Subtalar arthrodesis is performed through the (A) middle and (B) anterolateral portals. Calcaneocuboid arthrodesis is performed through the (C) lateral and (D) dorsolateral portals. Talonavicular arthrodesis is performed through the dorsolateral, (E) dorsomedial, and (F) medial portals. Plain radiographs 12 weeks post operative.

9. Technique for ankle arthroscopy

An understanding of the surface and intra-articular anatomy of the ankle region is essential to the successful performance of arthroscopy of the ankle. The superficial anatomy serves as a guide to the successful placement of arthroscopic portals in the ankle [13]. The neurovascular and tendinous structures are most at risk. Before portal placement, a skin marker is used to mark important anatomic landmarks, including the joint line, the dorsalis pedis artery, the greater saphenous vein, the tibialis anterior tendon, and the peroneus tertius tendon. The superficial peroneal nerve and its branches should be identified, if possible, because of their proximity to the anterolateral portal. These branches frequently can be seen, as they are pulled taut beneath the skin when the fourth toe is grasped and the forefoot is pulled into plantar flexion and adduction.

10. Setup and instrumentation

Arthroscopy of the ankle may be performed with general, regional, or local anaesthesia. The position of the patient may also vary, depending on the surgeon's preference. Supine placement of the patient is preferred, with the hip flexed 45 to 50 degrees on a non-sterile thigh holder. This supports the thigh proximal to the popliteal fossa. Adequate padding is added to avoid injury to the sciatic nerve [13]. An alternative method includes flexion of the knee over the end of the operating table with the patient supine. This permits some distraction by gravity and by an assistant. However, access to posterior portals is somewhat difficult with this technique [14].

Positioning the patient in the lateral decubitus position, with the body supported by a bean-bag & kidney rest and tilted posteriorly, has also been described [15]. This technique does not require the use of a thigh or ankle holder. For anterior portals, the ipsilateral hip is rotated externally; for posterolateral a portal, the hip is rotated internally [16]. Guhl [17] described the technique of placing the supine patient's ipsilateral hip & knee on a padded support. The foot and ankle are secured to an ankle holder, & a mechanical ankle distractor is used. A tourniquet may be used.

11. Ankle distraction

The decision to perform invasive or non-invasive distraction generally is made at the time of surgery and depends on both the laxity of the ankle joint and the location of the pathologic tissue that is to be addressed. With invasive distraction, a tibial pin and a talar or calcaneal pin are placed from the medial or lateral side with a mechanical distractor device. Non-invasive distractors include a clove-hitch-type device wrapped over the anterior aspect of the mid-foot & the posterior aspect of the heel (Figure. 11).

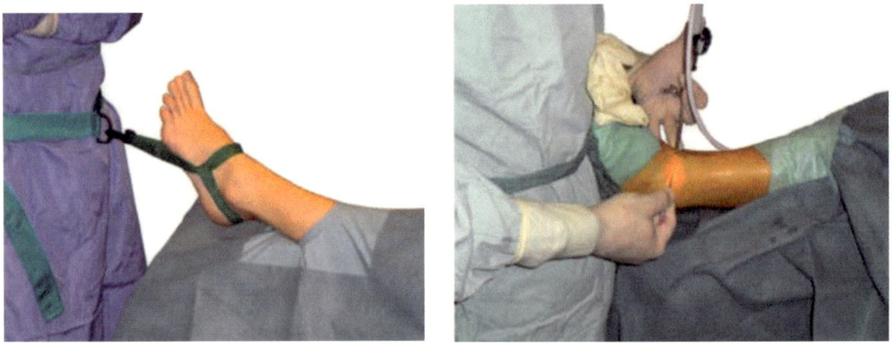

Figure 11. A resterilizable distraction device, which permits the surgeon to move the ankle quickly from the dorsiflexed position to the distracted position and vice versa.

12. Portal placement

Before portal placement, the ankle joint should be distended with 10 to 15 ml of lactated Ringer's solution injected into the ankle joint medial to the tibialis anterior tendon with the use of an 18- to 20-gauge needle. This injection also helps to establish the exact location of the anteromedial portal. Care should be taken to avoid directing the needle either too far anteriorly or too far posteriorly in the ankle joint. To prevent injury to neurovascular structures, the incisions for the portals should be made vertically and through the skin only. The deeper layers should be penetrated with a mosquito clamp followed by a blunt obturator, not with a sharp knife or a trocar. The anterolateral, anteromedial, and posterolateral portals are most commonly used. In a recent anatomic study [19] they were found to be the safest areas for portal placement, allowing no penetration of neurovascular structures.

12.1. Anteromedial portal

This is made just medial to the tendon of the tibialis anterior at, and just proximal to, the joint line (Figure 12, A). This portal is made first because it is easy to establish and is located in a region devoid of any major neurovascular structures. With the use of a blunt trocar, the arthroscope is carefully introduced into the joint. The portal is, on average, 9 mm lateral to the greater saphenous vein and 7.4 mm lateral to the greater saphenous nerve [3].

12.2. Anterolateral portal

The anterolateral portal is used for placement of the inflow cannula and is established under direct visualization with the use of a 25-gauge 1.5-inch needle. It is usually made just lateral to the tendon of the peroneus tertius at, or just proximal to, the level of the joint line. However, its location is also determined on the basis of the type and location of the pathologic tissue. This portal can sometimes be determined more easily by transilluminating the skin with the arthroscope to assist in the avoidance of neurovascular structures and tendons. The branches of the superficial peroneal nerve are most at risk. The mean distance of the anterolateral portal from the intermediate branch of the superficial peroneal nerve is 6.2 mm (range, 0 to 24 mm) [19].

12.3. Anterocentral portal

This may be created between the tendons of the extensor digitorum communis, at the level of the joint or proximal to the joint line. Care must be taken to avoid injury to the dorsalis pedis artery and the deep branch of the peroneal nerve, which lies between the extensor hallucis longus tendon and the medial border of the extensor digitorum communis tendon. Use of this portal is discouraged because of the inherent risk of neurovascular injury. Feiwell and Frey [19] found that the average distance (in either direction) of the portal from the artery, vein, and nerve is 3.3 mm (range, 0 to 10 mm).

12.4. Posterolateral portal

This is established just lateral to the Achilles tendon, approximately 1.0 to 1.5 cm proximal to the distal tip of the fibula (Figure 12, B). The portal can be made under direct visualization by placing the arthroscope from the anteromedial portal through the *notch of Harty*, looking posteriorly. An 18- gauge spinal needle is inserted just lateral to the Achilles tendon at a 45-degree angle toward the medial malleolus. The posterior aspect of the capsule is usually punctured just medial to the transverse tibio-fibular ligament.

An alternative for placement of the posterolateral portal is to place a switching stick (a smooth metal rod) from the anteromedial portal. The switching stick is inserted through the capsule, and the cannula is placed over the rod through the posterolateral portal. This can be done only with marked distraction of the joint. If the joint is not distracted sufficiently, this portal may be established too far proximally. The lesser saphenous vein and the sural nerve are at risk in establishing this portal. These two structures run parallel to each other along the posterolateral aspect of the ankle joint, an average of 3.5 mm apart. The sural nerve is consistently posterior to the lesser saphenous vein. On average, the posterolateral portal is 6 mm (range, 0 to 12 mm) posterior to the sural nerve and 9.5 mm (range, 2 to 18 mm) posterior to the lesser saphenousvein [19].

12.5. Postero-central portal

This portal is made just below the joint line through the middle of the Achilles tendon. This portal is not recommended because of its limitations and potential associated morbidity.

12.6. Posteromedial portal

This is generally contraindicated because of the proximity of the posterior tibial artery and nerve. The flexor hallucis and flexor digitorum longus tendons are also at risk, along with branches of the calcaneal nerve.

12.7. Transmalleolar portal

This portal may be necessary to drill osteochondral lesions of the talus. These portals are made by creating small incisions over the medial or lateral malleolus. A small-joint drill guide is helpful in directing the tip of the Kirschner wire to the lesion. Transtalar portals can be used by drilling from the sinus tarsi or the medial talus.

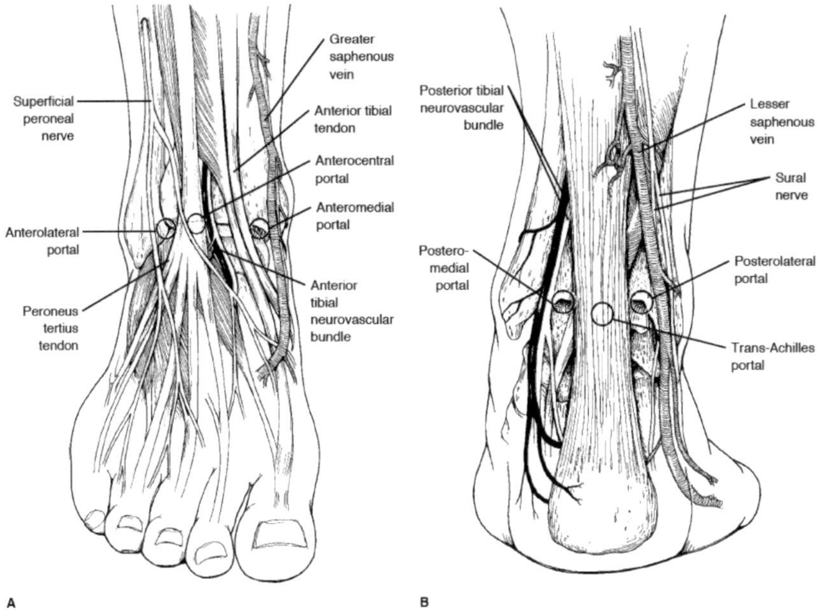

Figure 12. A, Location of the anteromedial, anterolateral, and anterocentral portals. The central portal should be avoided. **B,** The posterolateral portal is established just lateral to the Achilles tendon.

13. Arthroscopic examination

A 21-point arthroscopic examination enables the surgeon to perform a thorough, systematic evaluation of all areas of the ankle (Table 4) [20]. The use of this system allows reproducible documentation of the arthroscopic findings and accurate diagnosis of any intra-articular pathologic changes. In addition, it guarantees that all areas of the ankle joint are carefully inspected and provides a complete videotape record that can be reviewed in the future for both patient care and clinical studies of the patient population undergoing ankle arthroscopy.

The arthroscopic examination is always done initially through the anteromedial portal and subsequently through the anterolateral and posterolateral portals (Figure 13). Occasionally, one can slip out of the posterior capsule just enough to look down the sheath of the flexor

http://dx.doi.org/10.5772/54013

hallucis longus tendon as it runs in its groove on the posterior talus. Extreme caution is necessary to avoid injury to this structure.

Anterior	Central	Posterior
Deltoid ligament	Medial tibia and talus	Posteromedial gutter
Medial gutter	Central tibia and talus	Posteromedial talus
Medial talus	Lateral tibiofibular or talofibular articulation	Posterocentral talus
Central talus & overhang	Posterior inferior TFL	Posterolateral talus
Lateral talus	Transverse ligament	Posterior talo-fibular articulation
Trifurcation of the tibia/ talus/ fibula	Reflection of the flexor hallucis longus	Posterolateral gutter
Lateral gutter		Posterior gutter
Anterior gutter		

Table 4. 21-Point Arthroscopic Examination of the Ankle

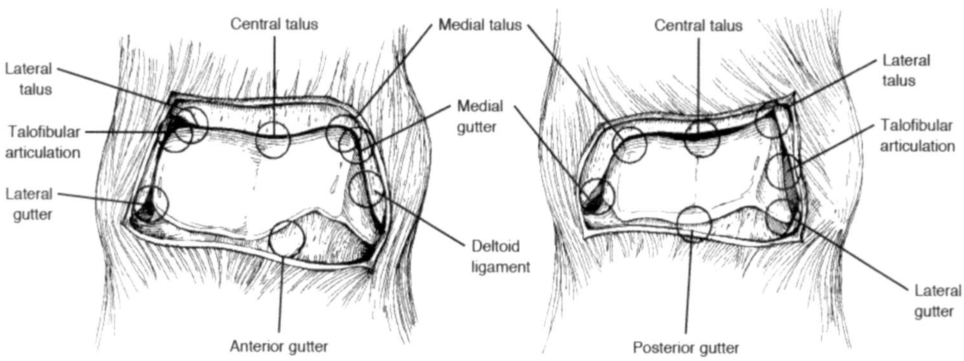

Figure 13. Left, The eight-point anterior examination of the ankle through the arthroscope. Right, The seven-point posterior examination

14. Complications

There are many potential complications with ankle arthroscopy (Table 4). Most can be avoided if the surgeon becomes thoroughly familiar with the surface anatomy of the region. Careful preoperative planning and the use of appropriate distraction and instrumentation techniques also help in avoiding complications.

In a series of 612 cases, Ferkel et al [21] found an overall complication rate of 9%. Neurologic complications were the most common (49%). In the 27 instances of neurologic injury, the superficial branch of the peroneal nerve was involved in 15 (56%); the sural nerve in 6 (22%); the greater saphenous nerve in 5 (18%); and the deep peroneal nerve in 1 (4%). In the same study, Ferkel et al also reported neurologic and arterial damage with the use of the antero-central or posteromedial portal, as well as with the use of distraction pins. The invasive distractor was used in 317 of 612 cases. Distraction pins were associated with some transient pin-tract pain, which resolved in all cases. No ligament injuries occurred in the ankle, but two stress fractures in the tibia occurred early in the series, when the pins were placed too far anteriorly or posteriorly in the tibia. One stress fracture occurred when the pin was placed in the fibula.

Ferkel et al also found superficial wound infection in six patients, which appeared to be related to the closeness of portal placement, the type of cannula used, early mobilization, and the use of tapes to close the portals. Deep wound infection occurred in two patients and was correlated with a lack of preoperative antibiotic therapy. Other complications included instrument failure, ligament injury, and incisional pain (two cases of each). Increased experience of the surgeon was associated with a lower complication rate. Compartment syndrome has not been reported in association with ankle arthroscopy. Some fluid extravasation occurs in all cases. The thinness of the skin and the lack of subcutaneous tissues around the ankle joint make postoperative swelling common. This usually responds well to elevation, compression, and application of ice. Thrombophlebitis and reflex sympathetic dystrophy can occur postoperatively, as they can after all operative procedures.

Overall, complications can be avoided by careful preoperative planning, meticulous surgical technique, the use of suitable small-joint instrumentation, and appropriate postoperative care (Table 5). It is mandatory to have a thorough understanding of the intra and extra-articular anatomy of the ankle and foot. In addition, practicing on plastic bone models and cadaver specimens can be particularly helpful in developing experience with small joint instrumentation and surgical procedures.

• Missed diagnosis	• Haemarthrosis
• Tourniquet complications	• Postoperative effusion
• Neurovascular injury	• Reflex sympathetic dystrophy
• Tendon injury	• Fluid-management complications
• Ligament injury	• Distraction-related complications (E.g., skin necrosis, pin problems)
• Wound complications	
• Infection	• Intra-operative fracture
• Articular cartilage damage	• Postoperative stress fracture
• Compartment ischemia	• Instrument breakage
• Compartment syndrome	

Table 5. Potential Complications of Ankle Arthroscopy.

http://dx.doi.org/10.5772/54013

15. Conclusion

Orthopaedic surgeons are always searching for ways to improve on current methods so as to provide maximal benefit for each intervention while minimizing its impact. Such benefits have been anticipated with ankle arthroscopy and in some instances have been realized. Compared with open arthrotomy, arthroscopy has the potential to shorten recovery times and limit surgical morbidity.

When used for the appropriate indications, ankle arthroscopy appears to give a high percentage of good results. Further refinement of techniques is necessary, and long-term comparative studies are needed to fully evaluate the efficacy of certain treatment protocols. Ankle arthroscopy should not replace a careful history and physical examination, an appropriate diagnostic workup, and a regimen of conservative therapy. The scope of arthroscopy and endoscopy of the foot and ankle is expanding. With sound knowledge regarding the indications, merits, and potential risks of new techniques, they will be powerful tools in foot and ankle surgery.

Author details

Jami Ilyas

Department of Orthopaedics, Royal Perth Hospital, Perth. Western Australia, Australia

References

[1] Burman MS. Arthroscopy of direct visualization of joints. An experimental cadaver study. J Bone Joint Surg 1931;13:669- 695.

[2] Watanabe M. Selfoc-Arthroscope (Watanabe no. 24 arthroscope). Monograph. Tokyo: Teishin Hospital, 1972.

[3] Feder KS, Schonholtz GJ: Ankle arthroscopy: Review and long-term results. Foot Ankle 1992; 13:382-385.

[4] Ferkel RD, Karzel RP, Del Pizzo W, et al: Arthroscopic treatment of anterolateral impingement of the ankle. Am J Sports Med 1991; 19:440-446.

[5] Liu SH, Raskin A, Osti L, et al: Arthroscopic treatment of anterolateral ankle impingement. Arthroscopy 1994; 10:215-218.

[6] Scranton PE Jr, McDermott JE: Anterior tibiotalar spurs: A comparison of open versus arthroscopic debridement. Foot Ankle 1992; 13:125-129.

[7] Ogilvie-Harris DJ, Mahomed N, Demazire A: Anterior impingement of the ankle treated by arthroscopic removal of bony spurs. JBJS Br 1993; 75:437-440.

[8] Ferkel RD, Scranton PE Jr: Arthroscopy of the ankle and foot. J Bone Joint Surg Am 1993; 75:1233-1242.

[9] Loomer R, Fisher C, Lloyd-Smith R, et al: Osteochondral lesions of the talus. Am J Sports Med 1993; 21:13-19.

[10] Myerson MS, Quill G: Ankle arthrodesis: A comparison of an arthroscopic and an open method of treatment. Clin Orthop 1991; 268:84-95.

[11] Ogilvie-Harris DJ, Lieberman I, Fitsialos D: Arthroscopically assisted arthrodesis for osteoarthrotic ankles. J Bone Joint Surg Am 1993; 75:1167-1174.

[12] Parisien JS, Shaffer B: Arthroscopic management of pyarthrosis. Clin Orthop 1992; 275:243-247.

[13] Ferkel RD: Arthroscopy of the ankle and foot, in Mann RA, Coughlin MJ (eds): Surgery of the Foot and Ankle, 6th ed. St Louis: Mosby, 1993, vol 2, pp 1277-1310.

[14] Andrews JR, Previte WJ, Carson WG: Arthroscopy of the ankle: Technique and normal anatomy. Foot Ankle 1985; 6:29-33.

[15] Parisien JS, Vangsness T: Operative arthroscopy of the ankle: Three years' experience. Clin Orthop 1985; 199:46-53.

[16] Parisien JS: Arthroscopic treatment of osteochondral lesions of the talus. Am J Sports Med 1986; 14:211-217.

[17] Guhl JF: Foot and Ankle Arthroscopy, 2nd ed. Thorofare, NJ: Charles B. Slack, 1993.

[18] Yates CK, Grana WA: A simple distraction technique for ankle arthroscopy. Arthroscopy 1988; 4:103-105.

[19] Feiwell LA, Frey C: Anatomic study of arthroscopic portal sites of the ankle. Foot Ankle 1993; 14:142-147.

[20] Ferkel RD: Arthroscopic Surgery: The Foot and Ankle. Philadelphia: Lippincott- Raven (in press).

[21] Ferkel RD, Guhl JF, Heath DD: Neurological complications of ankle arthroscopy: A review of 612 cases. Presented at the 13th Annual Meeting of the Arthroscopy Association of North America, Orlando, Fla, April 29, 1994.

[22] Close JR. Some applications of the functional anatomy of the ankle joint. J Bone Joint Surg [Am] 1987; 69-A: 596-604.

[23] Inman VT. The joint of the ankle. Baltimore: Williams and Wilkins, 1976.

[24] Ramsey PL, Hamilton W. Changes in tibiotalar area of contact caused by lateral talar shift. J Bone Joint Surg [Am] 1976; 58-A: 356-7.

[25] Choi WJ, Lee JW, Han SH, et al. Chronic lateral ankle instability: The effect of intra-articular lesions on clinical outcome. Am J Sports Med 2008; 36: 2167-2172.

[26] Ferkel RD, Chams RN. Chronic lateral instability: Arthroscopic findings and long-term results. Foot Ankle Int 2007; 28: 24-31

[27] DiGiovanni BF, Fraga CJ, Cohen BE, et al. Associated injuries found in chronic lateral instability. Foot Ankle Int 2000; 21: 809-815.

[28] Parisien JS, Shaffer B: Arthroscopic management of pyarthrosis. Clin Orthop 992; 275: 243-247.

[29] Meyer JM, Hoffmeyer P, Savoy X: High resolution computed tomography in the Chronically painful ankle sprain. Foot Ankle 1988; 8:291-296.

[30] Stetson & Ferkel, Ankle Arthroscopy: Indications & Results.J Am Acad Ortho Surg 1996;4:24-34

Chapter 2

Tibial Spine Avulsion Fractures: Current Concepts and Technical Note on Arthroscopic Techniques Used in Management of These Injuries

Vikram Sapre and Vaibhav Bagaria

Additional information is available at the end of the chapter

http://dx.doi.org/10.5772/54967

1. Introduction

Avulsion fractures of tibial spine, leading to discontinuity of anterior cruciate ligament fibers has been well described in literature in both pediatric and adult population. These fractures are also called as tibial eminence fractures or ACL avulsion fractures. They represent a variant of anterior cruciate ligament injury. Poncet in 1895 was probably the first person to document these types of injuries and it was only in 1959 that Meyers and McKeever described an account of surgical management of type II injuries of tibial spine. These injuries are commonly seen in children aged between 8-13 years and are usually sports related injuries occurring especially during cycling and skiing [1-3].In adults these injuries are commonly related to high energy trauma usually road traffic accidents [31] and have high incidence of associated injuries. The cause of increased incidence amongst children is hypothesized as being secondary to relative weakness of incompletely ossified tibial eminence compared to native ACL fibres [4].It has also been proposed that injury occurs secondary to greater elasticity of ligaments in young people [5].

2. Relevant anatomy

Tibial eminence is anatomically the eminent confluence of the medial and lateral plateaus and contains two spines. The medial spine bears the broad attachment of the ACL. The broad insertion of ACL fans out from the tibial eminence and coalesces with the attaching fibers of the anterior horn of medial meniscus anteriorly and the anterior horn of the lateral meniscus posterolaterally. The anatomy of these attachments also known as transverse intrameniscal ligament is important as they may get interposed between the fracture bed and the fractured fragment thereby preventing a successful reduction.

2.1. Classification

Mayer and Mc Keevers first described the method of classification in their article in 1959 [2].They classified these fractures based on degree of displacement of avulsed fragment.

- *Type I* fracture is an undisplaced fracture of tibial eminence, where in the avulsed fragment is not displaced from the fracture crater.
- *Type II* fracture is partially displaced fracture, in which the anterior part of the avulsed fragment is displaced superiorly from the bone bed and gives a beak like appearance on the lateral x-rays.
- *Type III* fracture is completely displaced fracture and there is no contact of avulsed fragment to the bone bed. Type III has been further subdivided into IIIA and B.
- *Type III* involves only ACL insertion and
- *Type III B* involves entire Intercondylar eminence.
- *Type IV* was later added by Zariczynj [8] to include comminuted fractures of tibial spine.

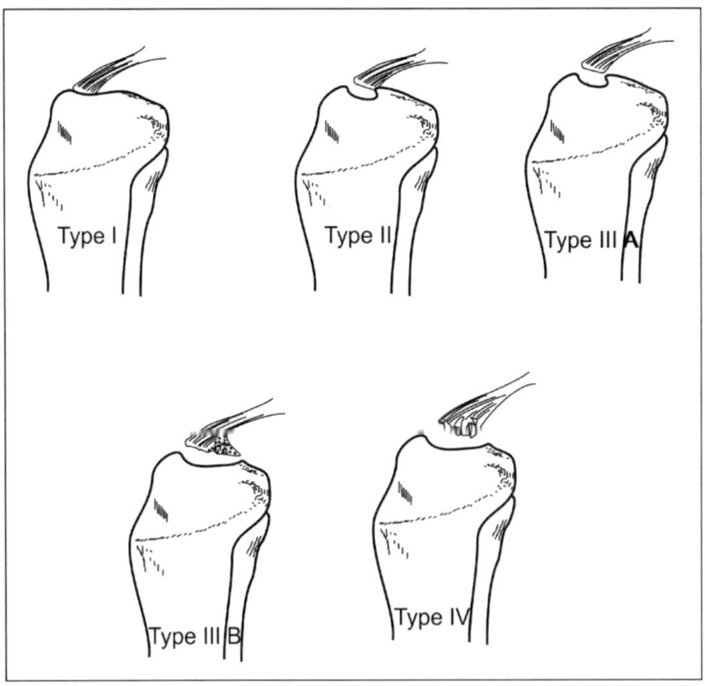

Figure 1. Mayer and Mc Keevers classification of tibial spine avulsion fracture. Type IV Comminuted fracture was added later by Zariczynj

http://dx.doi.org/10.5772/54967

2.2. Imaging

Standard imaging for tibial spine fractures include anteroposterior(AP) and lateral radiographs. Lateral radiographs should be true lateral radiographs which are particularly useful to assess degree of displacement and type of fracture. In skeletally immature patients the actual size of fragment may be significantly larger than what they appear on a radiograph owing to presence of cartilage in the fragment. A notch view is sometimes useful to better visualize the fragment in an AP plane. CT scan is useful in better assessment of fracture anatomy and degree of communition [9, 14]. MRI is useful in outlining the non-osseous concomitant injuries like meniscal injury, cartilage injury and other ligamentous injury [10, 11].

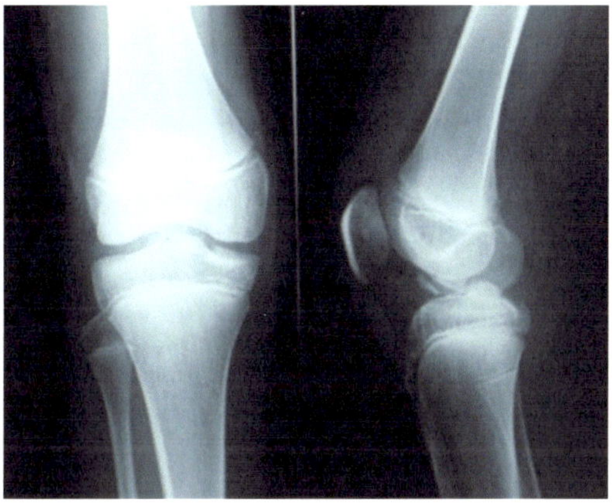

Figure 2. Anteroposterior and lateral view of tibial spine avulsion fracture in immature skeleton

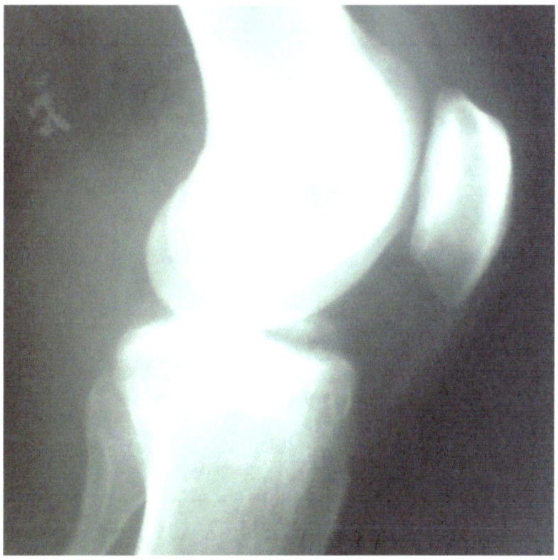

Figure 3. Lateral view of tibial spine avulsion fracture in mature skeleton

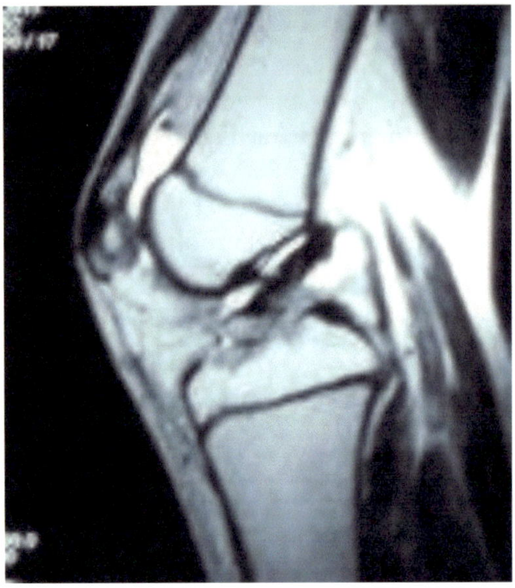

Figure 4. MRI of knee showing tibial spine avulsion fracture in immature skeleton

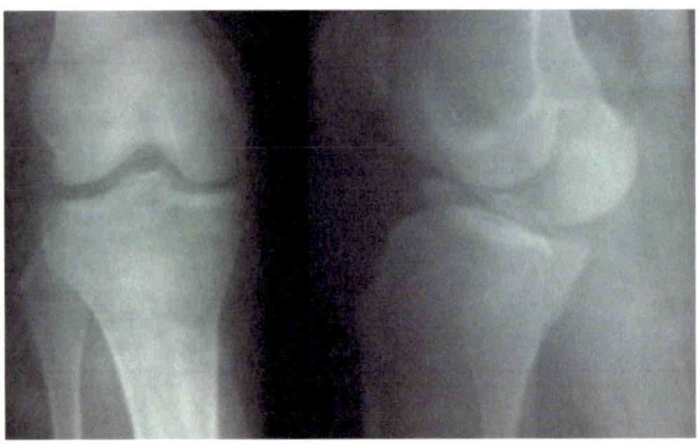

Figure 5. Radiograph of knee showing tibial spine avulsion fracture in Mature skeleton

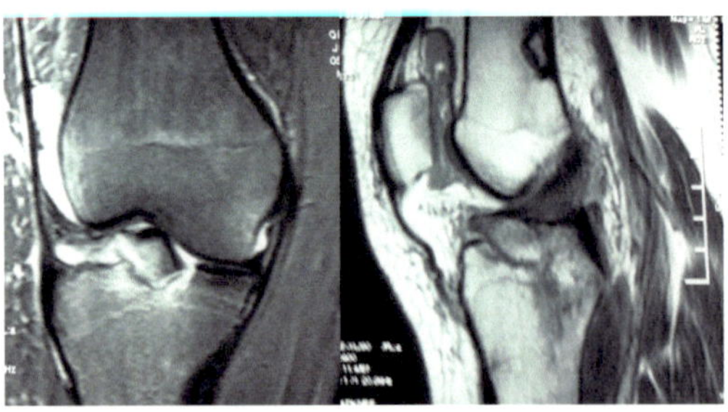

Figure 6. MRI of knee showing tibial spine avulsion fracture in Mature skeleton

2.3. Treatment

Treatment of tibial spine fractures depends on type of fracture, entrapment of soft tissues at fracture site and associated knee injuries.

Chief goals in treating tibial spine avulsion [12-16] are:

- Anatomical reduction of displaced fragment and achieving continuity of ACL fibers. While removing any block to reduction like bone fragments, blood clots, intermeniscal ligament or meniscus.
- Adequate rigid fixation which allows early range of motion exercises
- Eliminate the extension block and impingement due to displaced fragments

2.4. Type I

Type 1 fractures are treated with long leg cast immobilization for a period of 4-6 weeks. Radiographs are done immediately post immobilization to ensure that fragment is not displaced. Follow-up radiographs are done 2 weekly until 6 weeks. Position of knee immobilization in varying angles of flexion, extension and hyperextension has been described in the literature [2, 17]. There is no consensus amongst the researchers as to what should be the knee position during immobilization. We prefer to immobilize in full extension for a period of 4-6 weeks. Hyperextension stretches posterior neurovascular structures and hence should be avoided. Aggressive rehabilitation is required post immobilization to prevent knee stiffness.

2.5. Type II

Treatment of type II fractures has been controversial. In most cases closed reduction and immobilization may be attempted after aspirating knee haemarthrosis. Knee extension allows femoral condyles to reduce the displaced fragment. If acceptable reduction is achieved conservative management should be continued. Loss of reduction is common after conservative management of Type II fractures and should be closely monitored [18].If there is persistent superior displacement of the fragment seen on lateral radiographs then it is preferable to do arthroscopic reduction and internal fixation because there are high chances that there might be soft tissue entrapment at the fracture site.

2.6. Type III /IV

Treatment of displaced tibial spine avulsion fractures has evolved over a period of time from conservative management to open reduction and internal fixation to arthroscopic reduction and internal fixation. Various methods of fixation are used in operative treatment of these fractures varying from retrograde wires [8] /screws [26], antegrade screws [19],sutures [20, 21, 22, 23, 42],suture anchors [24], and a recently described suture bridge [44] and K wire and tension band wiring [25] technique.

There are only few comparative studies in literature to recommend which is the best technique of fixation for these fractures. Seon and Park [27] did a clinical comparative study of screw fixation and suture fixation method for tibial spine avulsion fractures and concluded that there is no significant clinical difference in terms of clinical outcome and stability. Bong and coworkers [28]in their biomechanical comparative study of screw versus fibrewire fixation concluded that fibrewire fixation was significantly stronger than cannulated screw fixation. Biomechanical comparison of 4 different methods of fixation was done by Mahar and collegues [29] on immature bovine knees. They concluded that 2 single-armed #2 Ethibond sutures, 3 bio absorbable nails, a single resorbable screw, or a single metal screw do not have any significant mechanical advantage over other. Tsukada [30] and coworkers did a biomechanical comparative study of antegrade screw fixation, retrograde screw fixation, and pullout suture fixation. They compared the initial fixation strength in response to a cyclic tensile load and found that antegrade screw is most effective in providing initial fixation strength.

2.7. Surgical technique–Pull through suture method

Patient is placed supine with affected leg secured on a leg holder. Standard arthroscopic setup and instruments are required for the surgery. Few instruments, which are specific to suture fixation technique, are 90-degree suture lasso with wire loop (Arthrex), epidural needle no.16 and suture retriever. Though image intensifier is not usually required it should be kept ready so that whenever it is required intraoperatively it can be used.

After giving IV antibiotics leg is exsanguinated and tourniquet is inflated. Standard antero-medial (AM) and anterolateral (AL) portals are made, adequate lavage is given to drain hematoma and clear the vision. The organized hematoma at the fracture site is removed with aggressive shaver blade and fat pad is removed if required. In all cases calf should be palpated at regular interval of time to assess compartment pressure.

Diagnostic arthroscopy is carried out assess additional injuries like meniscal injury, chondral injury or other ligament tears. Fracture crater is adequately cleaned, additional cancellous bone can be curetted to achieve better reduction. After achieving temporary reduction of fragment with 2mm kirschner wire from superomedial portal assess the reduction. Entrapped soft tissue or intermeniscal ligament are released if they are hindering the reduction.

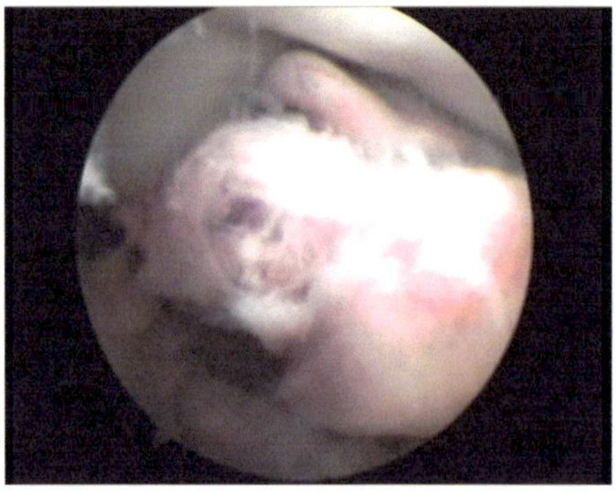

Figure 7. Avulsed fragment of tibial eminence

http://dx.doi.org/10.5772/54967

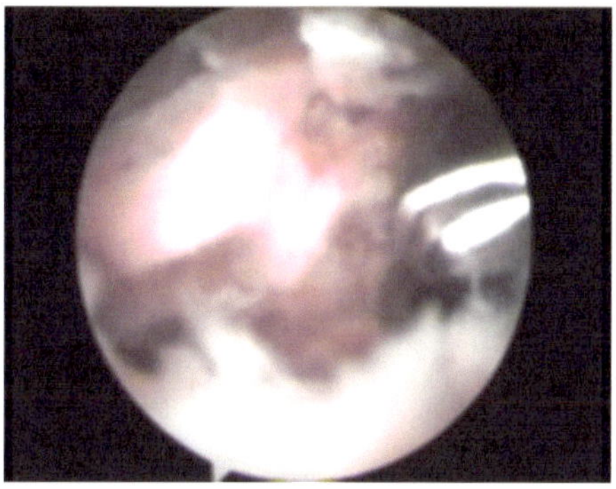

Figure 8. Avulsed fragment of tibial eminence being debrided with shaver

Two drill holes are made with 2.7 mm guide wire with the help of tibial ACL jig medial and lateral to anterior cruciate ligament (ACL) and exiting out on medial tibial cortex. With the scope in lateral portal and 90 degree suture lasso through medial portal a bite is taken in posterior half of ACL substance as close to fragment as possible and retrieve the cable loop through accessory lateral portal or by slightly enlarging lateral portal. Pass a fiber wire no. 2 through the loop and take it out through medial portal. This step is repeated by taking a suture bite through anterior half of substance of ACL.

Epidural or spinal needle no.16 is passed through medial tibial drill hole. Once epidural needle is seen in joint no.1 prolene loop is passed through the needle for suture shuttle. Prolene loop is retrieved through the medial portal. Both the fibrewire threads are passed through the prolene loop outside the joint and then prolene is pulled after holding lateral end of fibre wire with hemostat. Both fibre wire medial sutures will be shuttled through the medial tibial tunnel. This step is repeated for lateral sutures also and retrieved through lateral tibial tunnel.

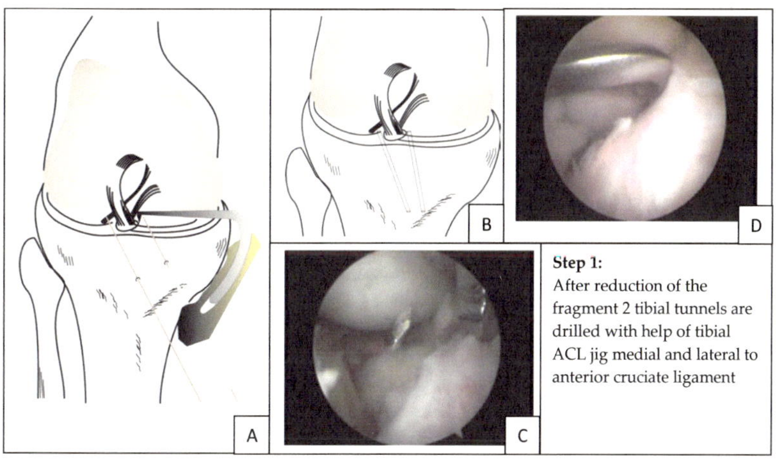

Figure 9. A,B,C,D: Formation of medial and lateral tibial tunnels

Both ends of fibre wire are held under traction and reduction is assessed. In full extension roof impingement is checked.If there is no obstruction to full extension sutures are tied independently over the bone bridge or if bone bridge is inadequate sutures can be tied over endobutton or suture wheel in extension.

In skeletally immature individuals tibial tunnels are made only through epiphysis. Entrance of the drill tip is confirmed under image intensifier before making tibial tunnels. Growth plate is not damaged with this method of fixation.

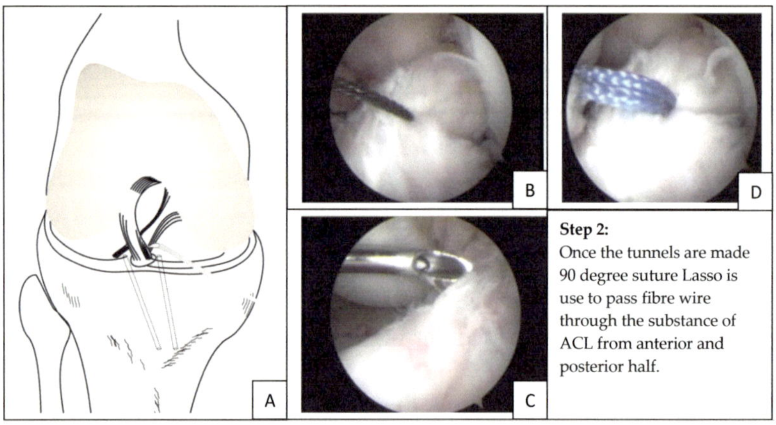

Figure 10. A,B,C,D: passage of lasso loop through the substance of ACL and exchanged with suture

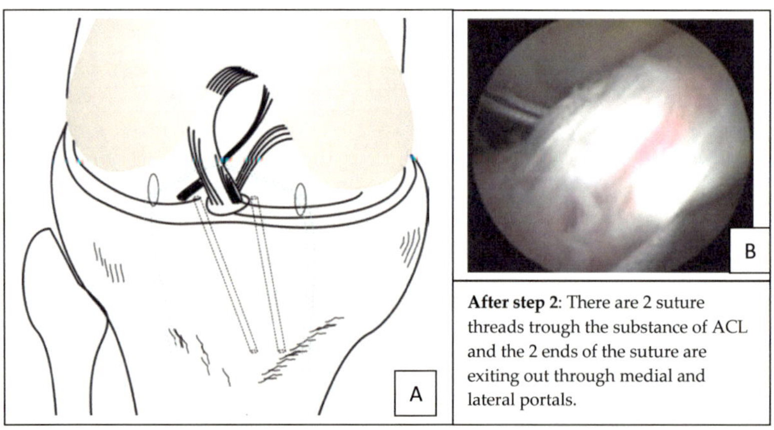

Figure 11. A,B: 2 sutures through the substance of ACL

http://dx.doi.org/10.5772/54967

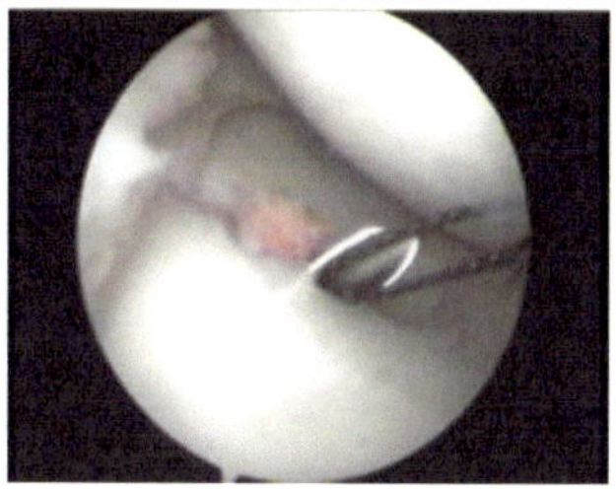

Figure 12. Lasso loop seen through spinal needle passed from one of tibial tunnels

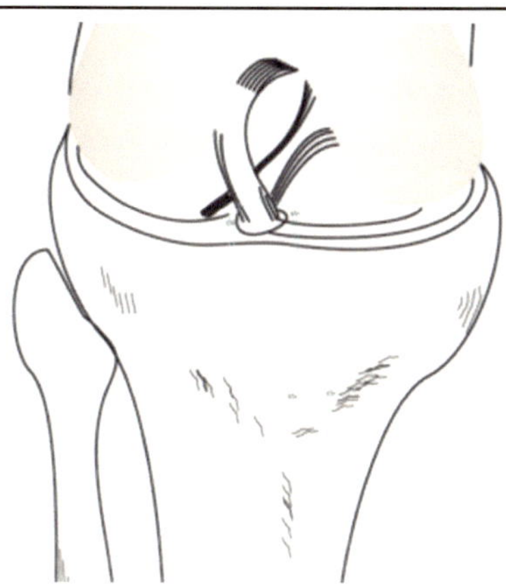

Figure 13. Sutures are seen passing from substance of ACL through tibial tunnels and final tightening is done over suture bridge

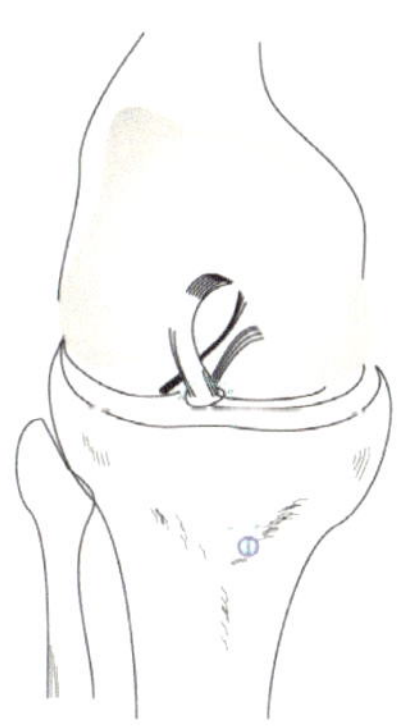

Figure 14. Lasso loop passed through the substance of ACL is tied over a suture disc, alternatively it can be tied over the bone bridge.

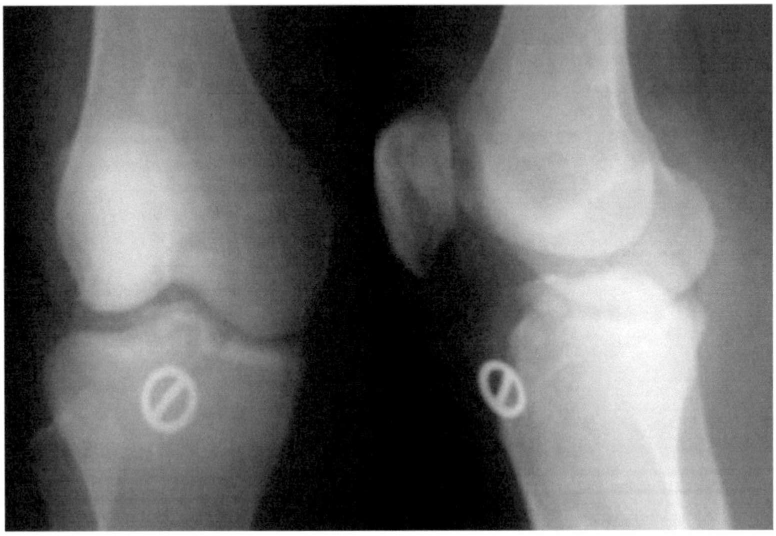

Figure 15. Post-operative X-ray showing reduction using pull through suture technique.

Suture fixation is preferable for comminuted fractures. Few authors have recommended suture fixation for all cases due to less risk of neurovascular involvement and less problem of implant prominence [12, 32]

2.8. Screw fixation

Patient is placed under supine position with affected leg on leg holder after administering general or regional anesthesia. Leg is exsanguinated after applying tourniquet.

Standard AM and AL portals are made and knee is adequately lavaged to clear the vision. Arthroscopic shaver is used to resect fat pad and organized hematoma at the fracture site.

Once the fracture site has been debrided reduction is attempted with ACL guide or 90 degree chondroplasty awl. In case intermeniscal ligament hinders the reduction and also cannot be mobilized resection is performed.

After achieving temporary reduction a guide wire from 4mm cannulated cancellous (C.C) screw is inserted through superomedial portal to temporarily hold the reduction. Reduction and guide wire placement is confirmed under image intensifier. This temporary fixation guide wire can be used for screw fixation or an additional wire under image guidance can be introduced. Cannulated cancellous drill bit is drill hole 4mm screw. 4 mm cc screw of appropriate length which is just holding the posterior cortex is used for fixation. Placement of screw is confirmed under image. A second screw can also be placed in provisional fixation wire if fragment is large enough.

Once adequate fixation is done guide wires are removed and knee is gently moved through gentle range of motion. Terminal extension is verified and arthroscopically assessed for notch impingement.

http://dx.doi.org/10.5772/54967

For skeletally immature individuals guide wire is stopped before entering the tibial physis. Drilling is done under image guidance to avoid crossing the tibial physis. Screw length should be just short of tibial physis.

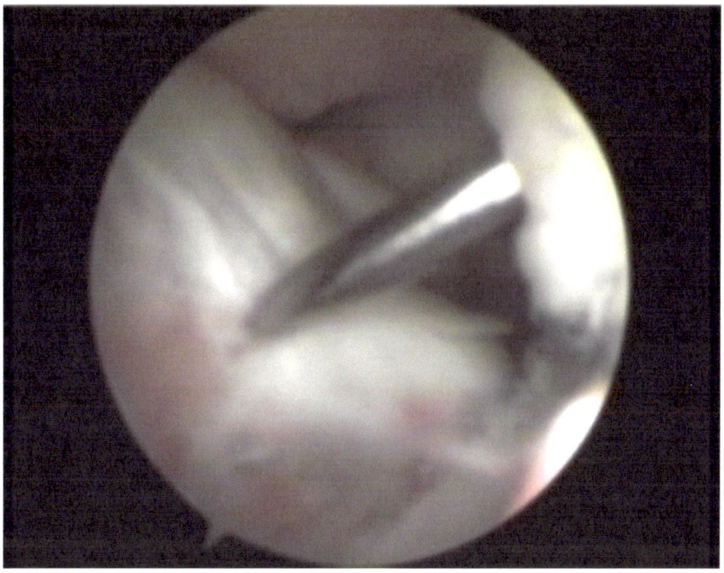

Figure 16. Temporary fixation achieved through guide wire passed from superomedial portal

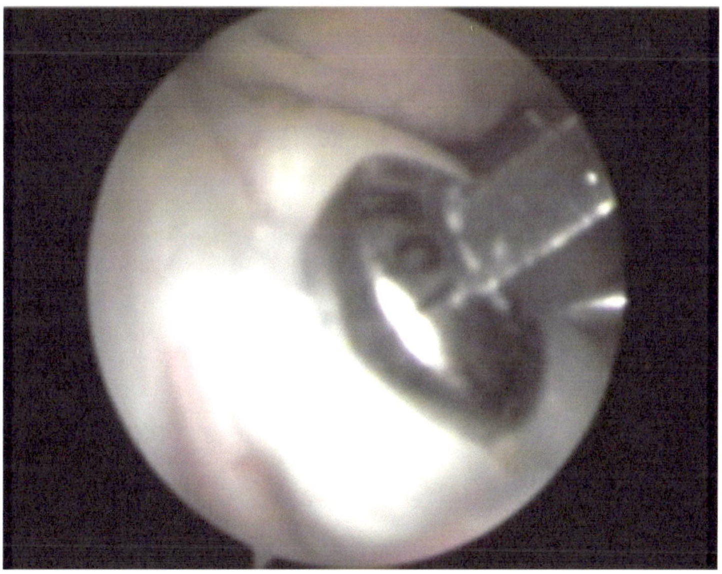

Figure 17. Screw fixation achieved for avulsed fragment

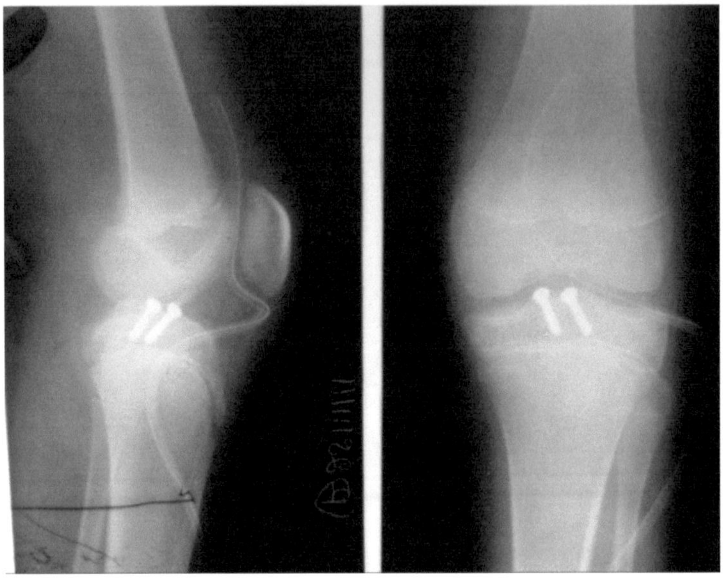

Figure 18. Screw fixation post op x-rays

3. Post–operative rehabilitation

Tibial eminence fractures have excellent prognosis. Previously, prolonged immobilization may lead to arthrofibrosis and a permanent loss of full extension. Therefore, earlier rehabilitation is crucial as it encourages a faster recovery and prevents the development of secondary complications [33]. Rehabilitation is similar to ACL tear protocols activities include static cycling, leg presses, elastic theraband or tubing exercises [34]. Patient is allowed to bear weight through a pair of elbow crutches and as per tolerance. Initial phase include closed kinetic chain exercise like heel slides on bed for ROM and static quads, heel press and SLR in long knee brace. As weight bearing improves, partial squats are included for gaining strength. Studies show that proprioceptive training plays important role in ACL rehabilitation [35-37]. Initial exercise includes balance on rocker board progressed to balance on wobble board. This can further be complicated with tossing the ball between the therapist and the patient while the patient balances himself on the wobble board. After achieving grade four of muscle strength, agility training like zigzag running, karoke, figure of eight running, hops, etc can be incorporated. Along with training of lower limb muscles emphasis is also given on core strengthening exercises.

4. Complications

Main complications associated with tibial spine avulsion fractures are residual laxity, arthrofibrosis, implant prominence and growth deformity in pediatric patients.

Residual laxity [38] is most common complication of tibial spine avulsion fractures in both conservative and operative method of treatment. Despite the presence of residual laxity most patients are clinically asymptomatic [38, 39].Few authors have recommend countersinking of the fragment to decrease the residual laxity [38, 40].

Arthrofibrosis results due to prolonged immobilization following a conservative treatment or malunion of the fragment [41]. Aggressive rehab protocol is advised after operative treatment of these fractures to prevent arthrofibrosis. While doing arthroscopic reduction and internal fixation it is recommended to assess the notch in extension to rule out notch impingement and inadequate reduction which can lead to extension loss.

Hardware prominence is common with screw fixation device. Hardware prominence can lead to notch impingement and extension loss. For symptomatic implant prominence implant removal is treatment of choice.

Growth disturbance after fixation of these fractures is uncommonly seen. It is recommended for patients with immature skeleton to undergo physis sparing fixation method [42, 43].

5. Conclusion

Tibial spine avulsion injuries are frequently seen by arthrosocopic surgeons. It is important that they are diagnosed promptly. Various treatment options exist and generally the results are good if an anatomic reduction is obtained.

Author details

Vikram Sapre[1] and Vaibhav Bagaria[2]

1 NKP Salve Institute of Medical Sciences and Research Centre, Nagpur, India

2 Care Hospital, Nagpur & ORIGYN Clinic, India

References

[1] Gronkvist, H. Fracture of the anterior tibial spine in children. J Pediatr Orthop, (1984). , 4, 465-468.

[2] Meyers, M. H, & Mckeever, F. M. Fracture of the Intercondylar eminence of the tibia. J Bone Joint Surg Am (1959). , 41, 209-222.

[3] Meyers, M. H, & Mckeever, F. M. Fracture of the intercondylar eminence of the tibia. J Bone Joint Surg Am (1970). , 52, 1677-1683.

[4] Wiley, J. J, & Baxter, M. P. Tibial spine fractures in children. ClinOrthop Rel Res, (1990)., 255, 54-60.

[5] Noyes, F. R, Delucas, J. L, & Torvik, P. J. Biomechanics of anteriorcruciate ligament failure: An analysis of strain-rate sensitivity and mechanism of failure in primates. J Bone Joint Surg Am(1974)., 56, 236-253.

[6] Markatos K, Kaseta MK, Lallos SN, Korres DS, Efstathopoulos NThe anatomy of the ACL and its importance in ACL reconstruction.Eur J OrthopSurgTraumatol. 2012

[7] Siegel L, Vandenakker-Albanese C, Siegel DAnterior cruciate ligament injuries: anatomy, physiology, biomechanics, and management.Clin J Sport Med. 2012 Jul;22(4): 349-55

[8] Zaricznyj, B. Avulsion fracture of the tibial eminence treatedby open reduction and pinning. J Bone Joint Surg Am (1997)., 59, 1111-1114.

[9] Griffith, J, Antonio, G. E, Tong, C. W, et al. Cruciate ligament avulsion fractures. Arthroscopy (2004)., 20(8), 803-12.

[10] Toye, L, Cummings, P, & Armendariz, G. Adult tibial intercondylar eminence fracture:evaluation with MR imaging. Skeletal Radiol (2002)., 31(1), 46-8.

[11] Prince, J, Laor, T, & Bean, J. MRI of anterior cruciate ligament injuries and associated findings in the pediatric knee: changes with skeletal maturation. AJR Am J Roentgenol (2005)., 185(3), 756-62.

[12] Lubowitz, J. Part II: arthroscopic treatment of tibial plateau fractures: Intercondylar eminence avulsion fractures. Arthroscopy (2005)., 21(1), 86-92.

[13] Hunter, R. E, & Willis, J. A. Arthroscopic fixation of avulsion fractures of the tibialeminence: technique and outcome. Arthroscopy. (2004). Feb;, 20(2), 113-21.

[14] Griffith, J, Antonio, G. E, Tong, C. W, et al. Cruciate ligament avulsion fractures. Arthroscopy (2004)., 20(8), 803-12.

[15] Medler, R, & Jansson, K. Arthroscopic treatment of fractures of the tibial spine. Arthroscopy (1994)., 10(3), 292-5.

[16] Seon, J, Park, S. J, Lee, K. B, et al. A clinical comparison of screw and suture fixation of anterior cruciate ligament tibial avulsion fractures. Am J Sports Med (2009)., 37(12), 2334-9.

[17] Fyfe, I. S, & Jackson, J. P. Tibial intercondylar fractures in children: a review of the classification and the treatement of malunion. Injury (1981)., 13, 165-169.

[18] Mclennan, J. G. Lessons learned after second-look arthroscopy in type III fractures of the tibial spineJ Pediatr Orthop. (1995). Jan-Feb;, 15(1), 59-62.

[19] Reynders, P, Reynders, K, & Broos, P. (2002). Pediatric and adolescent tibial eminence fractures: arthroscopic cannulated screw fixation. J Trauma , 53(1), 49-54.

[20] Ahn, J. H, & Yoo, J. C. (2005). Clinical outcome of arthroscopic reduction and suture for displace acute and chronic tibial spinefractures. Knee Surg Sports Traumatol Arthrosc , 13(2), 116-121.

[21] Lehman RA Jr, Murphy KP, Machen MP, Kuklo TR ((2003). Modified arthroscopic suture fixation of a displace tibial eminencefracture. Arthroscopy 19(2):E6

[22] Su, W. R, Wang, P. H, Wang, H. N, & Lin, C. J. modified arthroscopic suture fixation of avulsion fracture of the tibial Intercondylar eminence in children. J Pediatr Orthop B , 20, 17-21.

[23] Medlar, R. G, & Jansson, K. A. Arthroscopic treatment of fractures of the tibial spine. Arthroscopy (1995). , 11, 328-331.

[24] Vega, J. R, Irribarra, L. A, Baar, A. K, Iniguez, M, Salgado, M, & Gana, N. (2008). Arthroscopic fixation of displaced tibial eminence fractures: a new growth plate-sparing method. Arthroscopy Knee Surg Sports Traumatol Arthrosc. A new procedure for tibial spine avulsion fracture fixation Matthew A. Mann Nicholas M. Desy Paul A. Martineau, January 2012, 24(11), 1239-1243.

[25] Yudong Gan, Dachuan Xu, Jing Ding and Yongqing Xu Knee Surg Sports Traumatol Arthrosc.Tension band wire fixation for anterior cruciate ligament avulsion fracture: biomechanical comparison of four fixation techniques(2012). , 20(5), 909-915.

[26] Van Loon, T, & Marti, R. K. A fracture of the intercondylar eminence of the tibial treated by arthroscopic fixation. Arthroscopy (1991). , 7, 385-388.

[27] Seon, J, Park, S. J, Lee, K. B, et al. A clinical comparison of screw and suture fixation of anterior cruciate ligament tibial avulsion fractures. Am J Sports Med (2009). , 37(12), 2334-9.

[28] Bong, M, Romero, A, Kubiak, E, et al. Suture versus screw fixation of displaced tibial eminence fractures: a biomechanical comparison. Arthroscopy (2005). , 21(10), 1172-6.

[29] Mahar, A, Duncan, D, Oka, R, et al. Biomechanical comparison of four different fixation techniques for pediatric tibial eminence avulsion fractures. J Pediatr Orthop (2008). , 28(2), 159-62.

[30] Tsukada, H, Ishibashi, Y, Tsuda, E, et al. A biomechanical comparison of repair techniques for anterior cruciate ligament tibial avulsion fracture under cyclic loading. Arthroscopy (2005). , 21(10), 1197-201.

[31] Kendall, N, Hsy, S, & Chan, K. Fracture of the tibial spine in adults and children. A review of 31 cases. J Bone Joint Surg Br (1992). , 74(6), 848-52.

[32] Biyani, A, Reddy, N. S, Chaudhury, J, Simison, A. J, & Klenerman, L. The results of surgical management of displaced tibial plateau fractures in the elderly. Injury (1995).

[33] Accousti, W. K, & Willis, R. B. Tibial eminence fractures. Orthop Clin N Am (2003). , 34(3), 365-75.

[34] Roya Salehoun and Nima Pardisnia ((2007). Rehabilitation of tibial eminence fracture. Journal of Canadian Chiropratice association, 51(2).

[35] Griffin, L. Y. Rehabilitation of the injured knee. 2nd edition. Mosby (1995).

[36] Heijne, A, Fleming, B. C, Renstron, P. A, Peura, G. D, Beynnon, B. D, & Werner, S. Strain on the anterior cruciate ligament during closed kinetic chain exercises. Am Coll Sports Medicine (2004). , 36, 953-941.

[37] Nicholas, J. A, & Heshman, E. B. The lower extremity & spine in sports medicine. 2nd edition. Mosby (1995).

[38] Kocher, M, Foreman, E, & Micheli, L. Laxity and functional outcome after arthroscopic reduction and internal fixation of displaced tibial spine fractures in children. Arthroscopy(2003). , 19(10), 1085-90.

[39] Willis, R, Blokker, C, Stoll, T. M, et al. Long-term follow-up of anterior tibial eminence fractures. J Pediatr Orthop (1993). , 13(3), 361-4.

[40] In, Y, Kim, J. M, Woo, Y. K, et al. Arthroscopic fixation of anterior cruciate ligament tibial avulsion fractures using bioabsorbable suture anchors. Knee Surg Sports Traumatol Arthrosc (2008). , 16(3), 286-9.

[41] Vander Have KGanley TJ, Kocher MS, et al. Arthrofibrosis after surgical fixation of tibial eminence fractures in children and adolescents. Am J Sports Med (2010).

[42] Ahn, J, & Yoo, J. Clinical outcome of arthroscopic reduction and suture for displaced acute and chronic tibial spine fractures. Knee Surg Sports Traumatol Arthrosc(2005). , 13(2), 116-21.

[43] Mylle, J, Reynders, P, & Broos, P. Transepiphysial fixation of anterior cruciate avulsion in a child. Report of a complication and review of the literature. Arch Orthop-TraumaSurg (1993). , 112(2), 101-3.

[44] Matthew A. Mann, Nicholas M. Desy, Paul A. Martineau. A new procedure for tibial spine avulsion fracture fixation January 2012. Knee Surgery Sports Traumatology Arthroscopy.

Chapter 3

Lumbar Intervertebral Disc Endoscopy

Ștefan Cristea, Florin Groseanu,
Andrei Prundeanu, Dinu Gartonea, Andrei Papp,
Mihai Gavrila and Dorel Bratu

Additional information is available at the end of the chapter

http://dx.doi.org/10.5772/54544

1. Introduction

Unlike any other arthroscopic procedure this doesn't rely on the existence of a distension liquid or gaseous medium. In fact we visualize more or less bleeding regions that cannot be distended [6], [7].

The procedure is mini-invasive and it addresses to the herniated intervertebral lumbar disc.

Because of the evolution of the human species, the development of the vertebral curves, the standing position, the dehydration of the intervertebral disc, the degeneration processes following aging discal suffering occurs. The most frequent form is the lumbar herniated disc mainly located in the L4-L5 and L5-S1 motion segments [1], [3].

2. Anatomical features of the lumbar spine

2.1. Functional spinal unit (FSU) or motion segment

A functional spinal unit (FSU) is the smallest physiological motion unit of the spine to exhibit biomechanical characteristics similar to those of the entire spine (Fig. 1). A FSU consists of two adjacent vertebrae, the intervertebral disc and all adjoining ligaments between them and excludes other connecting tissues such as muscles. The intervertebral ligaments are (anterior to posterior): anterior longitudinal ligament, posterior longitudinal ligament, facet capsular ligaments, interspinous ligament, ligamentum flavum (yellow ligament), and supraspinous ligament.

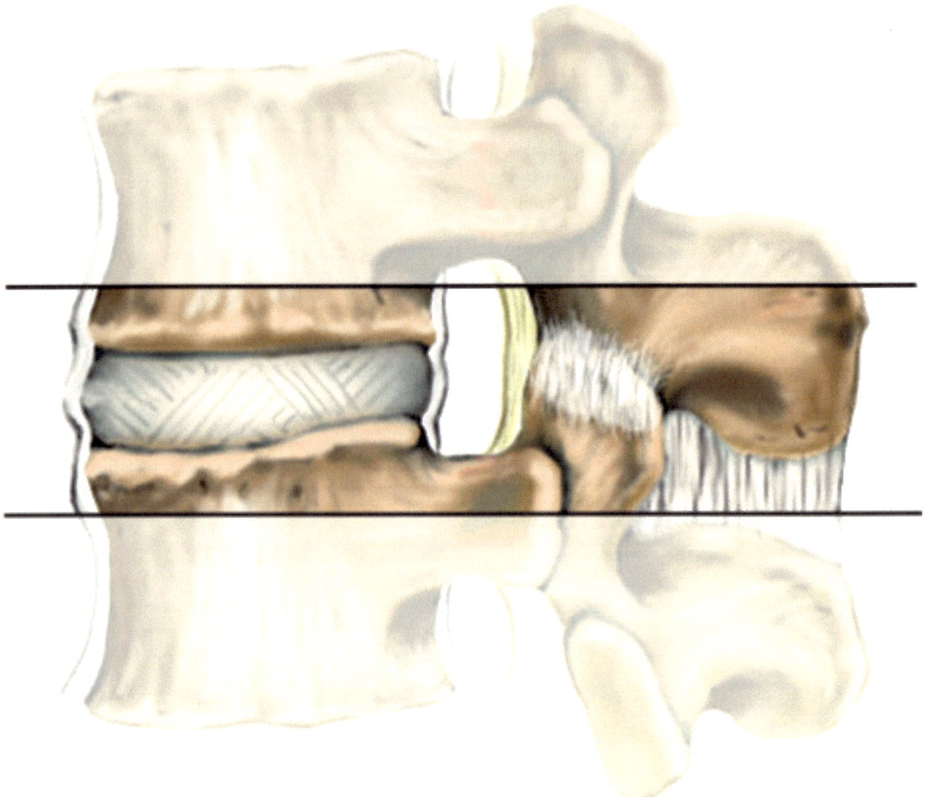

Figure 1. Motion segment (FSU) [1],[5],[11]

Another term for the FSU is spinal motion segment.

Each intervertebral motion segment displays the following movements:

- inclination of one vertebra to the other
- slip
- axial rotation.

So the movements are:

- Flexion – extension
- Axial rotation
- Lateral inclination left – right of one vertebra to the other

The motion segments are specialized for a certain type of motion, depending on the anatomical region. All the lumbar pieces realize 10^0-15^0 of axial rotation, 80^0 of flexion – extension, 30^0 of lateral inclination [2],[11].

http://dx.doi.org/10.5772/54544

The areas where the curves are reversed, where there are areas of different mobility are the election site of the traumatic lesions, especially in the lumbo-sacral region. Demand is very high in the L5 disc from the changing of the region of motion and curves – lumbar lordosis over the sacrococcigian piece kyphosis. The upper plateau of the sacrum is 30^0-60^0 inclined from horizontal. Lumbar lordosis curvature is quite opposite to the sacro-coccigian curvature. All the weight above the lumbosacral level is cushioned by the L5 disc and then successively gradually by L4, L3... These stresses are exacerbated naturally in human by standing and sitting positions. These are added to the repeated stresses by bending, weight lifting, falls from height. Gradually with age, biochemical changes occur, dehydration, responsible for degenerative lesions at these levels.

2.2. The intervertebral discs

The intervertebral discs in the lumbar region are at least 10 mm thick representing a third of the lumbar vertebral body height.

The vertebral discs form one of the anterior aspects of the vertebral foramen and as the spinal nerves pass through the foramen they are just behind the corresponding discs. In addition, the discs take part in the anterior wall of the vertebral canal thus any posterior herniation of the disc can compress the spinal cord and the corresponding spinal nerves.

Every disc is structurarely characterized by three structures: the central nucleus pulpous, the annulus fibrosus and the cartilaginous end plates. The disc is anchored to the vertebral body by the fibres or the annulus fibrosus and the cartilaginous endplates.

The nucleus pulpous consists of soft tissue, highly hydrophilic, placed in the centre of the disc. There is not a clear separation between the nucleus pulpous and the annulus fibrosus, the main difference being the density of the fibres, the nucleus having large extrafibrilar spaces with a highly glycosaminoglycan content which allows the water retention. The nucleus pulpous position varies from a region to other, being more posterior in the lumbar region. Its position is related with several functional aspects.

The nucleus pulpous consists of a tridimensional network of collagen fibres embedded in a highly hydrated proteoglycan containing gel. The loss of this proteoglycan gel with aging decreases the water content until, in the advanced degenerated discs, the total loss of proteoglycan. This is the major change accompanying the dehydration with age. At the beginning of life the water content is 80-88% and it deceases to 70% in the fourth decade. Loss of proteoglycan and matrix disorganization has other important mechanical effects; because of the subsequent loss of hydration, degenerated discs no longer behave hydrostatically under load.

The annulus fibrosus is located at the outer disc. This is made up of a series of concentric rings called lamellae, with the collagen fibers lying parallel within each lamella. The fibers are oriented at approximately 30^0 to the horizontal axis, alternating to the left and to the right of it in adjacent lamellae, thus resulting in a 120^0 change in angle between plans (Fig. 2). These have a special role, with different tensioning, in the mobility and determine an increased resistance. The structure is similar to a tire sustaining high forces of compression, torsion and traction [1], [5], [11].

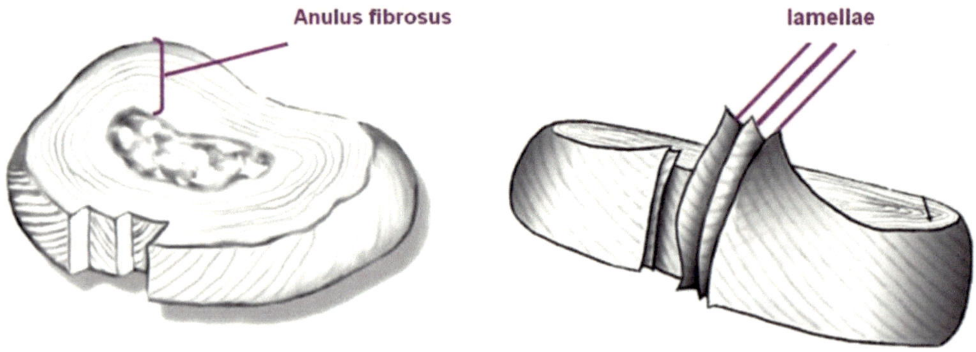

Figure 2. Intervertebral disc structure [1],[5],[11]

The density of the fibro-cartilagineous lamellae varies according to the place in the annulus fibrosus, thus being denser anteriorily and posteriorly than on the lateral sides. The lamellae do not form complete circles, but they divide themselves or merge with each other to connect with other strips. The postero-lateral region of the annulus tends to be more irregular and less ordered. With age, the structure of the annulus becomes weaker in this area predisposing to the herniation of the nucleus.

Elastin fibers are also found in the composition of the nucleus pulpous and of the annulus firosus. In the annulus they are disposed circularly, obliquely and vertically.

The annulus attachment to the vertebrae is made by passing over the edges of the cartilage endplates and then goes up beyond the compact bone and the edges of adjacent vertebral body and its periosteum, forming stable connections between adjacent vertebral bodies. These perforating fibers are interwoven with fibrilar lamelae of trabecular bone.

According to Modic [10], the altered signal intensity detected by MR imaging is not, in and of itself, the causal pathologic process but rather a reflection of the causal process, which is some type of biomechanical stress or instability. A formal classification was subsequently provided by Modic et al in 1988 [10], based on a study of 474 patients, most of whom had chronic low back pain (LBP). These authors described 2 types of endplate and marrow changes: Type 1 changes were hypointense on T1-weighted imaging (T1WI) and hyperintense on T2-weighted imaging (T2WI) and were shown to represent bone marrow edema and inflammation (Fig.3).

Type 2 changes were hyperintense on T1WI and isointense or slightly hyperintense on T2WI and were associated with conversion of normal red hemopoietic bone marrow into yellow fatty marrow as a result of marrow ischemia (Fig.4).

http://dx.doi.org/10.5772/54544

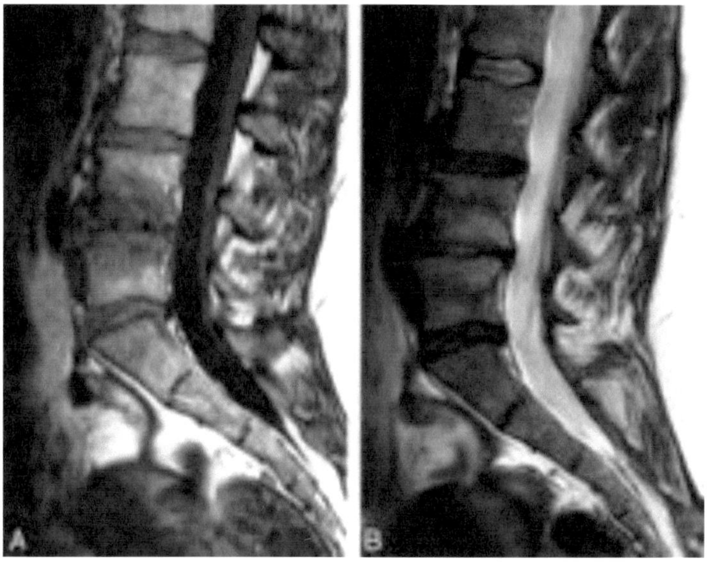

Figure 3. Modic type 1 changes are hypointense on T1WI (*A*) and hyperintense on T2WI (*B*).

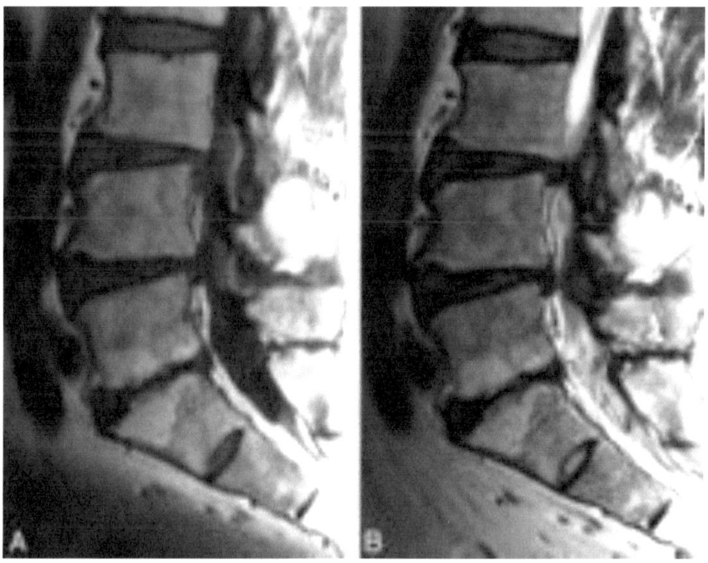

Figure 4. Modic type 2 changes are hyperintense on T1WI (A) and isointense or hyperintense on T2WI (B).

Modic type 3 changes were subsequently described as hypointense on both T1WI and T2WI and were thought to represent subchondral bone sclerosis. Mixed-type 1/2 and 2/3 Modic changes have also been reported, suggesting that these changes can convert from one type to another and that they all represent different stages of the same pathologic process. The absence of Modic changes, a normal anatomic appearance, has often been designated Modic type 0 (Fig.5).

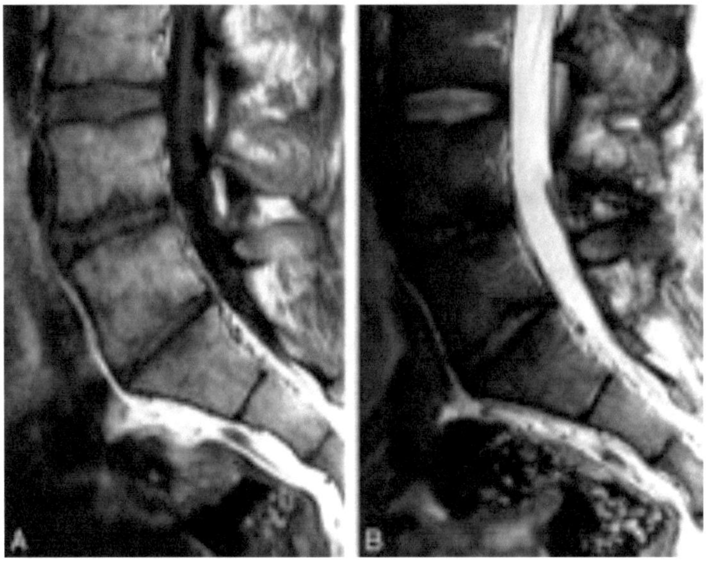

Figure 5. Modic type 3 changes are hypointense on both T1WI (*A*) and T2WI (*B*).

2.3. Ligaments

Vertebral bodies are secured together by the longitudinal ligaments that extend the whole length of the spine. The ligaments are multifunctional and bind the osseous pieces together. They protect the vertebral column and the nevrax from injuries. They are multilayered, composed of elastin and collagen fibers. Ligaments do not oppose compressive forces. They limit the range of every motion for not exceeding the physiological limits.

There are seven ligaments attached (Fig.6) to the motion segment:

1. Anterior longitudinal ligament
2. Posterior longitudinal ligament
3. Yellow ligament (ligamentum flavum)
4. Facet capsulary ligaments
5. Intertransverse ligament
6. Interspinous ligament
7. Supraspinous ligament

Degenerative ligament lesions reduce the range of motion between two adjacent vertebral pieces. On the other hand, excessive ligament tension may result in abnormal segmental movement as it happens in young gymnasts and acrobats. This abnormality can produce degenerative lesions, osteofites that can cause canal stenosys [1], [3], and [13].

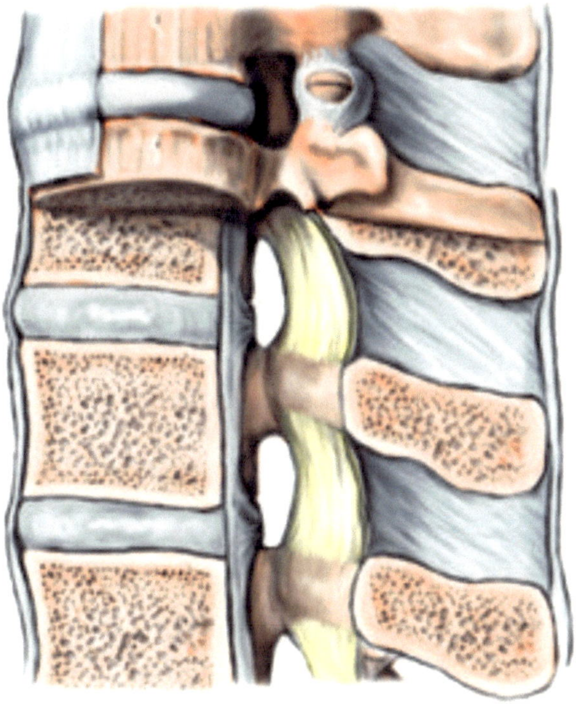

Figure 6. Motion segment ligaments [1],[5],[11]

2.4. Spinal nerve structures, Meninges

As part of the Central Nervous System (CNS), the spinal cord is located immediately below the brain stem and extends from the foramen magnum to L1.

At L1 the spinal cord terminates as the conus medularis. Below L1, the thick but flexible dural sac contains the spinal nerves collectively known as the cauda equina.

Also contained within the cauda equina is the filum terminale, which extends from the conus medularis to the coccyx and acts as an anchor to keep the lower spinal cord in its normal shape and position.

The individual nerve roots of the cauda equina are suspended in spinal fluid. At this level, it is possible to pass a needle safely into the thecal sac for evaluation of spinal fluid or injection of various materials such as drugs, anesthetics, or radiologic substances.

Within the spinal canal, the spinal cord is surrounded by the epidural space. This space is filled with fatty tissue, veins, and arteries. The fatty tissue acts as a shock absorber and keeps the spinal cord away from the bony tissue of the vertebrae.

The brain and spinal cord are covered by three layers of material called meninges. The main function of these layers is to protect and feed the delicate neurological structures (Fig. 7).

The dura mater is the outermost meningeal layer and is made up of strong connective tissue. The dura mater, also called the dura, is gray in color and is generally easy to identify within the spinal canal. The dura extends around each nerve root and becomes contiguous with the epineurum, a membrane covering the spinal nerves.

The subdural space is a very small space between the dura and the next meningeal layer, the arachnoid layer. The arachnoid layer is highly vascularized with a web of arteries and veins that give the impression of a spider web. It is thinner than the dura and is subject to injury.

Below the arachnoid layer is the subarachnoid space, which is filled with cerebrospinal fluid (CSF). The CSF helps to protect the nerve structures by acting as a shock absorber. It also contains various electrolytes, proteins, and glucose. A spinal tap can be inserted into the subarachnoid space to retrieve CSF for various chemical analyses.

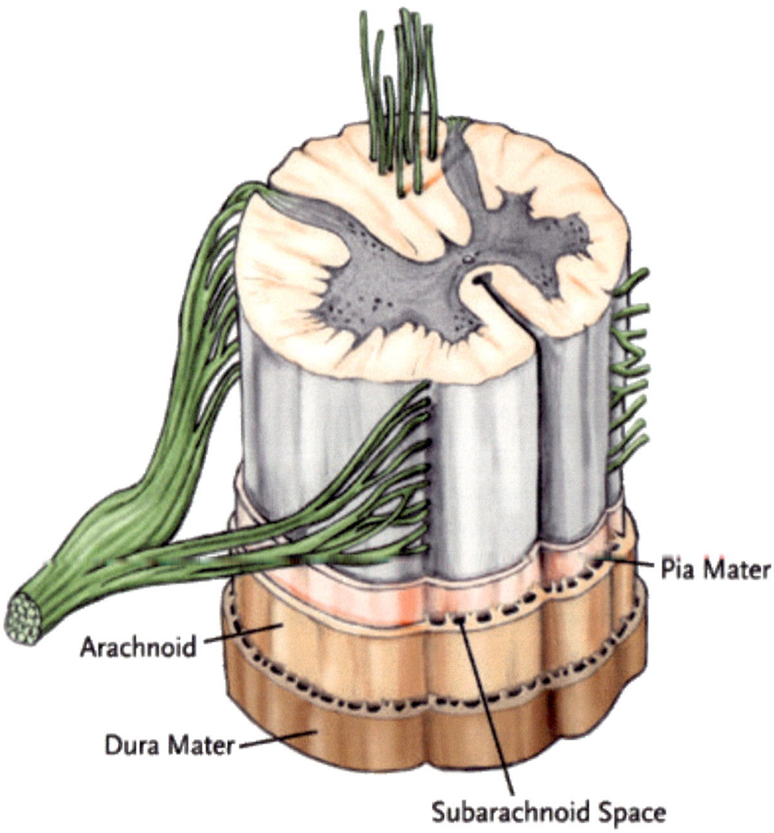

Figure 7. Meningeal structure [1],[5],[11]

The innermost lining of the meninges is called the pia mater. It is closely adhered to the spinal cord and the individual nerve roots. It is highly vascular and gives blood supplies to the neurological structures [1], [3], and [13].

2.5. Topography

There are 31 pairs of spinal nerves: 8 cervical, 12 thoracic, 5 lumbar, 6 sacrococcygeal. The first cervical nerve root exits between the skull (C0) and C1. The 8th cervical nerve root exits between C7 and T1. Thereafter, all nerve roots exit at the same level as the corresponding vertebrae. For example, the L1 nerve root exits between L1 and L2.

The nerve roots emerge from the spinal cord higher than their actual exit through the intervertebral foramen. This means that the spinal nerves must often pass downwards adjacent to the spinal cord before exiting through the intervertebral foramen. This leaves the nerves exposed to risk of compression by protruding disc material. Therefore, it is possible to have a compression of the L5 nerve root at the L4-L5 disc space.

Each spinal nerve root has both motor nerves and sensory nerves. Motor nerves conduct information and orders from the brain to the peripheral nervous system to excite a muscular contraction. Sensory nerves receive information from the periphery (skin, fasciae, tendons, ligaments, muscles) and send the information towards the brain.

Motor fibers are located on the anterior aspect of the spinal cord. Multiple filaments of motor fibers are called ventral roots or anterior roots. The cell bodies or control centers of the motor nerve roots are located within the spinal cord. Damage or injury to the anterior roots or motor cell bodies may result in the loss of musculoskeletal function.

Sensory fibers are located on the posterior aspect of the spinal cord. Each collection of sensory fibers is called a dorsal root or posterior root. The sensory nerves have a special accumulation of cell bodies called the dorsal root ganglia. The ganglia are the control centers of the sensory nerves and are located outside but close to the spinal cord. Just beyond the ganglia, the anterior and posterior roots become joined in a common dural sheath. It is at this point that the peripheral nerve is formed [4], [11].

2.6. Vascularization and innervations

The spinal column receives segmental arterial vascularization from the adjacent vessels: for the lumbar region from lumbar and iliolumbar arteries and for the pelvic region from lateral sacral arteries. All these branches anastomozes and give anterior and posterior spinal arteries that irrigate the marrow.

It is interesting that the intervertebral disc is a poorly vascularized structure. It receives nutrition by passive diffusion through the central vertebral endplates.

The vascularisation of the vertebral body is different in its structure. The most poorly vascularized region is adjacent to the disc. As we approach the central area it becomes more vascularized. The central region can be divided into a nutritive artery vascularized area and a metafizeal arteries vascularized area. The peripheric region is vascularized by short peripherial arteries. Oxygenation and metabilic feeding of the disc is regional and determines the lamelae and fibrous ring arrangement. Fluid located between the blades is channeled vertically. Frequent movement of blades may increase the diffusion. One of the aging concequences is arterial occlusion and diminished blood flow.

Diminished blood flow at the delicate lombar arteries, especially at the fifth pair, through aging and occlusion by dsc compresion, explains the degenerative pathology of the L5 disc.

The veins form communicative plexuses all along the spine. The plexuses drain in the lumbar and the lateral sacral veins. The internal vertebral plexuses form a continuous network between the dura mater and the vertebral canal walls. Two anterior branches, one on each side of the posterior longitudinal ligament make an anastomosis in front of the ligament and receive the bazivertebral vein. They are interconnected with the basilar and occipital sinuses. Internal posterior plexuses merge lamella and the yellow ligaments level. There are anterior and posterior communications between the internal and external plexuses.

The Azygos system comunicates with a valveless venous network known as Batson's plexus, or Crock veins (Fig.8). When the vena cava is partially or totally occluded, Batson's plexus provides an alternate route for blood return to the heart. Because of the azygos system, patient positioning is very important in posterior lumbar spine surgery. The patient's abdomen should always hang free and without abdominal pressure. An increase in pressure will diminish flow through the azygos system and the vena cava. This results in an increase of venous flow into Batson's plexus with a corresponding increase of blood loss. Furthermore, increased bleeding makes it difficult to visualize the spinal cord, nerve roots, and disc during surgery. The vessels of Batson's plexus may be referred to as epidural veins and are often cauterized during posterior interbody procedures. However, these vessels are difficult to identify and cauterize, even when there is no increased abdominal pressure.

Innervation of the intervertebral disc, ligament structures and fibrous connective tissue of the spinal canal, has great clinical importance. It is provided by a recurrent nerve, the sinuvertebral nerve. In many ways it can be considered equivalent to the recurrent meningeal branch of the cranial nerves. It has dual origin from spinal nerves and sympathetic system. The spinal part arises distal to the dorsal root ganglion and reenter the spinal canal reaching back into the median, then gives rise to discal branches, for the disc above and below. At the same time innervates the medial facet of te interapofizar joint capsule. C and A-δ fibers are involved in pain transmission, these structures explains the pain caused by compression of the anterior and posterior nerve fibers on the periphery of the ring [1],[4],[13].

2.7. Important anatomical related structures

It should be noted that the spinal cord ends at the disc between L1 - L2. Below this level is cauda equina (horse tail), covered by meninges to the S2.

Anterior to the lombar vertebrae are the large abdominal vessels – the aorta and vena cava.

The aorta bifurcates into the common iliac arteries at L4 level. Here also the origins of the middle sacral artery and branches of the iliolumbar artery from the internal iliac artery. These arteries irrigate L5 and the sacrococcygeal area.

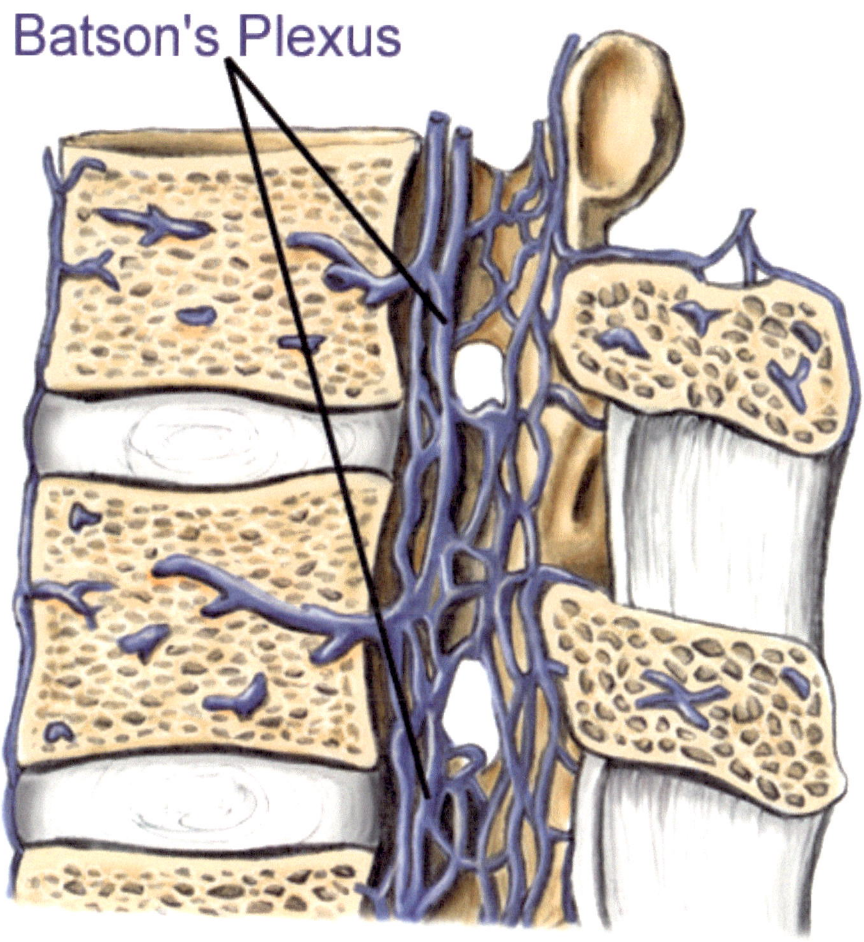

Figure 8. Venous vascularisation [1],[5],[11]

Vena cava originates at the level of L4, by the convergence of left and right common iliac vein. It is located on the right side of the spine, going through the abdomen and thorax to the heart. Common iliac veins results from internal and external iliac veins. The iliac veins can be injured during the anterior arthrodesis of L3-L4 and L4-L5. The common iliac veins are thick and strong but the iliac veins are thin and sinuous and special attention should be taken with the surgical gestures near them.

The endoscopic surgery must take account of these relationships because if the iliac vessels are damaged it is hard to obtain haemostasis. The surgery must be converted into a classical open one.

The second lumbar vertebrae have contact with the kidneys in the lateral-superior side and more anteriorly with the digestive tube.

At lumbar level the posterior paravertebral muscles are well represented and the thoraco-lumbar fascia is thick and strong.

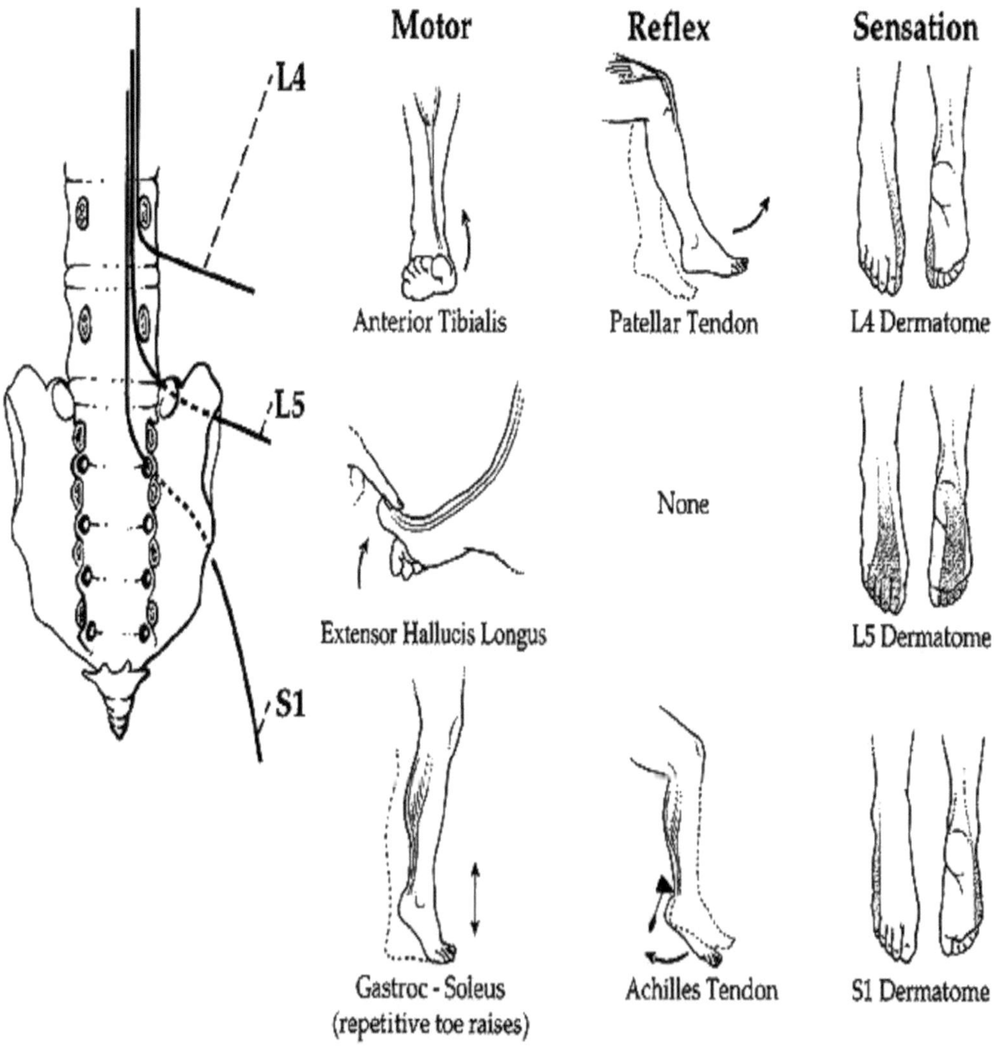

Figure 9. L4S1-Nerve roots

Endoscopic surgery must be performed only after complete and qualified clinical examination (Fig.9), followed by posterio-anterior and lateral view X-rays, CT and MRI exam with Modic [10] stage classification of the modified disc.

3. History

In 1934 Mixer and Barr accomplished the first discectomy by hemilaminectomy; in 1948 Ottolenghi preformed a vertebral puncture. The first decompression of the vertebral disc by dorsal approach was made by Kabin in 1973. In 1975 the first percutaneous nucleotomy was performed by Hihikata using fine cannulae. In 1976 Hj Leu accomplished the puncture of the disc by dorsolateral approach, using in the same manner two long and fine cannulae with trocar [5],[9],[12].

Our days the newly endoscopic device was developed based on the ordinary arthroscope with 0 degree telescope in 1994, by French neurosurgeon Jean Desandau [6],[7], on the principle of microsurgery, than taken over and improved by the Storz Company in 2004.

The first endoscopy of a lumbar disc hernia in Romania was performed in 2005 [5].

4. Indications for treatment [5], [6], [7]

Basically 90-95% of all disc lesions are successfully treated by conservatory means. Only 5-10 % of lesions who do not respond to conservative treatment will be surgically treated.

The conservative treatment is used between a minimum of 4-6 weeks and a maximum of 3-6 months. It consist of relative resting on a hard bed, flexing the hips and the knees for relaxation in hyperlordosis, administrating non steroidal anti-inflammatory drugs accompanied by gastric protection, muscle relaxers, anti-inflammatory and decontracting physiotherapy, epidural anaesthesia, and possible vertebral manipulations with the mechanical reinsertion of the disc.

The treatment is applied gradually, progressively, and after the decrease of pain we can try medical gymnastics for toning the paravertebral and abdominal muscles.

If the conservative treatment was applied correctly without a response from the patient, we will intervene more aggressively.

4.1. The surgical options are numerous:

- percutaneous discectomy
- chemonucleolysis using chemopapain
- automated percutaneous lumbar suction discectomy, like laser disc decompression – suction and intervertebral decompression, reducing the pressure will momentarily diminish the pain, followed by the aggravation of the degenerative symptoms, producing advanced

of arthrosis to the interapophyseal and intra-articular joints with the posterior segment actually bearing the overweight.

- Microscopic discectomy
- Intervertebral endoscopy
- radiofrequency techniques
- electrotermical interdiscal therapy
- limited laminectomy
- percutaneous intersomatic arthrodesis PLIF - TLIF - ALIF + BMP / growth factors + computer guided surgery
- artificial disc
- morfogenic biological Bone solutions protein BMP / growth factors

Technically the **surgical indications** are:

1. onset of sphincter disorders
2. paresis – motor weakness
3. increased conduction velocity of nerve root
4. the persistence/increased pain although it is properly treated for 4 weeks
5. recurrence of pain after a period of relief

5. Indications for lumbar disc endoscopy

Basically one can successfully intervene in any phase (subligamentar protrusive or extrusive or transligamentar) of discopathy without borders. Furthermore in the lumbar canal stenosis the canal can be endoscopically recalibrated even in cases of sequestration of the herniated disc, also for foraminal hernia.

Most authors perform a partial ablation of the herniated material, similarly to an arthroscopic meniscectomy.

The endoscopic approaches are:

- dorsal approach – the most popular
- ventral approach
- postero-lateral approach
- lateral approach

http://dx.doi.org/10.5772/54544

The dorsal endoscopic approach is derived from the intervertebral dorsal approaches for laminectomy performed by neurosurgeons and orthopaedists in the surgical treatment of the herniated disc.

The approach used is intraseptal paraspinous described by Wiltze in 1988. An interlaminar window is created through foraminectomy.

The equipment was developed based on the ordinary arthroscope with 0 degree telescope, by French neurosurgeon Jean Desandau [6], [7], on the principle of microsurgery, later improved by Storz Inc (Fig.10).

The surgeon's training should be complex and requires a learning curve.

Occasionally the discal endoscopy could be converted into classical surgery due to possible complications or for transpedicular stabilization.

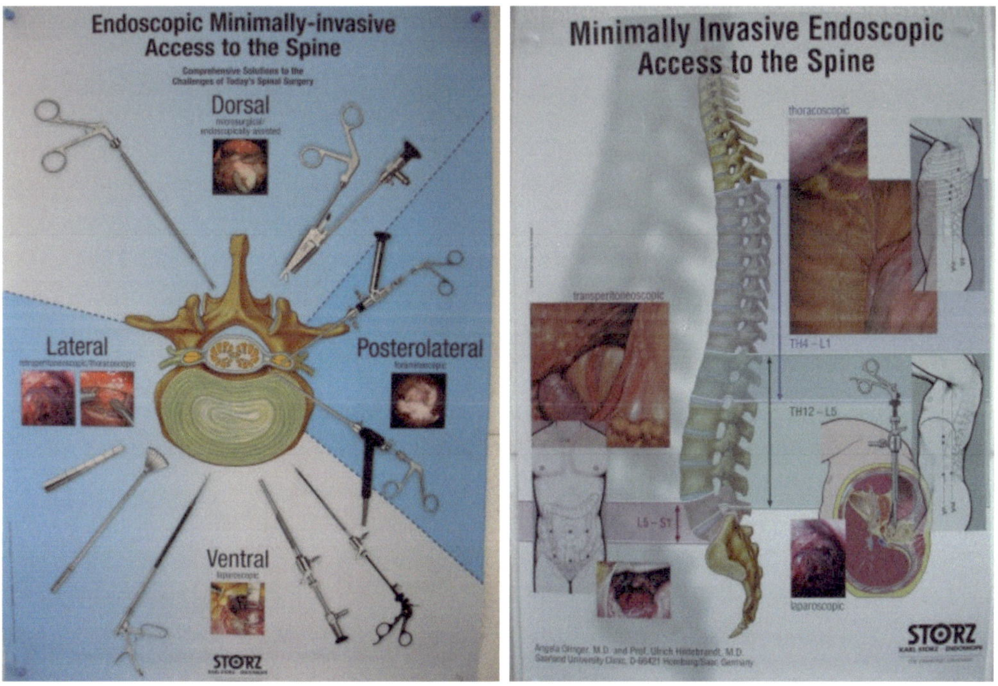

Figure 10. Endoscopic MIS approaches

5.1. Patient positioning

The patient under general anesthesia is in prone position on a radiotransparent surgical table. The level for the surgical approach is established by clinical and radiological criteria. Using special cushions the abdominal pressure is released, the cava pressure is released, the hips and the knees are in hyperflexion so that the intervertebral spaces are opened along with the hyperflexion of the lumbar spine. Thus the bone resection is kept to a minimum and the migrated disc can be reached (Fig11).

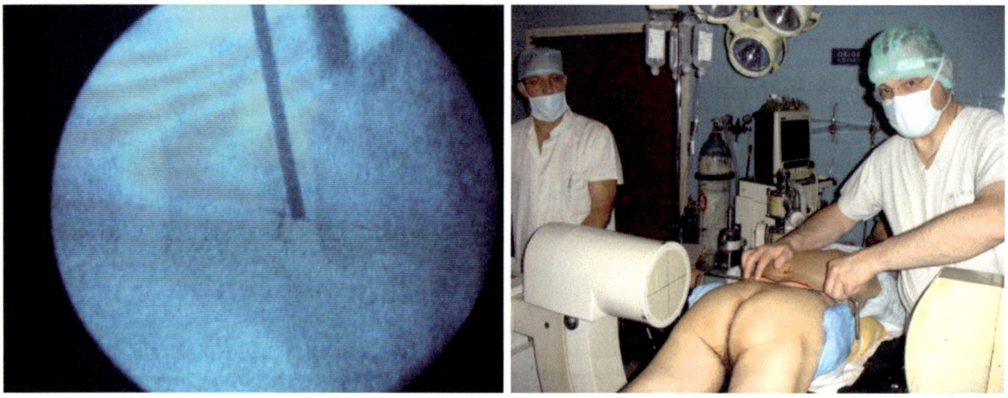

Figure 11. Fluoroscopic guidance – landmark of the level for the surgical approach

5.2. Surgical technique

The approach is similar to classic discal surgery. A local anesthetic is infiltrated to decrease bleeding. A paravertebral 3 cm incision is performed on the migrated disc's side, shown by the CT and MRI exams, followed by a lateral paravertebral muscle dissection. Haemostatic compresses are inserted at both end of the incision, a trocared speculum is inserted, deep to the vertebral plane then the trocar is removed and replaced with the optic component.(Fig 12 a,b,c,d)

A foraninectomy is performed and an interlaminary window is done.(Fig 12c,d). The nerve root is retracted (Fig 12 e,f) and released from the scar tissue, it is centrally reclined and the herniated disc is spotted. Discectomy is performed. (Fig 12 g,h)

The yellow ligaments are excised. The root is highlighted, and released from the scar tissue, it is centrally reclined and the herniated disc is highlighted. Disc ablation is performed. Some authors excise strictly the herniated, compressive material, others excise the entire disc but intersomatic fusion must be performed otherwise the forces become unbalanced, overloading the posterior arch. Hemostasis is performed with specially adapted bipolar forceps. The compresses are removed then fascia, aponeurosis and skin sutured and bandaged (Fig.12i).

Another posterior transforaminal technique with dilators (Fig. 13) with direct light was developed by Wolfe & Metronic. The surgical details are similar, but several dilatators are used.

In Switzerland, Dr. Leu imagined a more laborious technique by lateral approach, performing two mini-invasive lateral portals with special instruments, long and with small diameter. One portal is for visualizung and the other is the working portal. Low efficiency, high price and additional risks decreased the practice of this lateral technique (Fig.14).

http://dx.doi.org/10.5772/54544

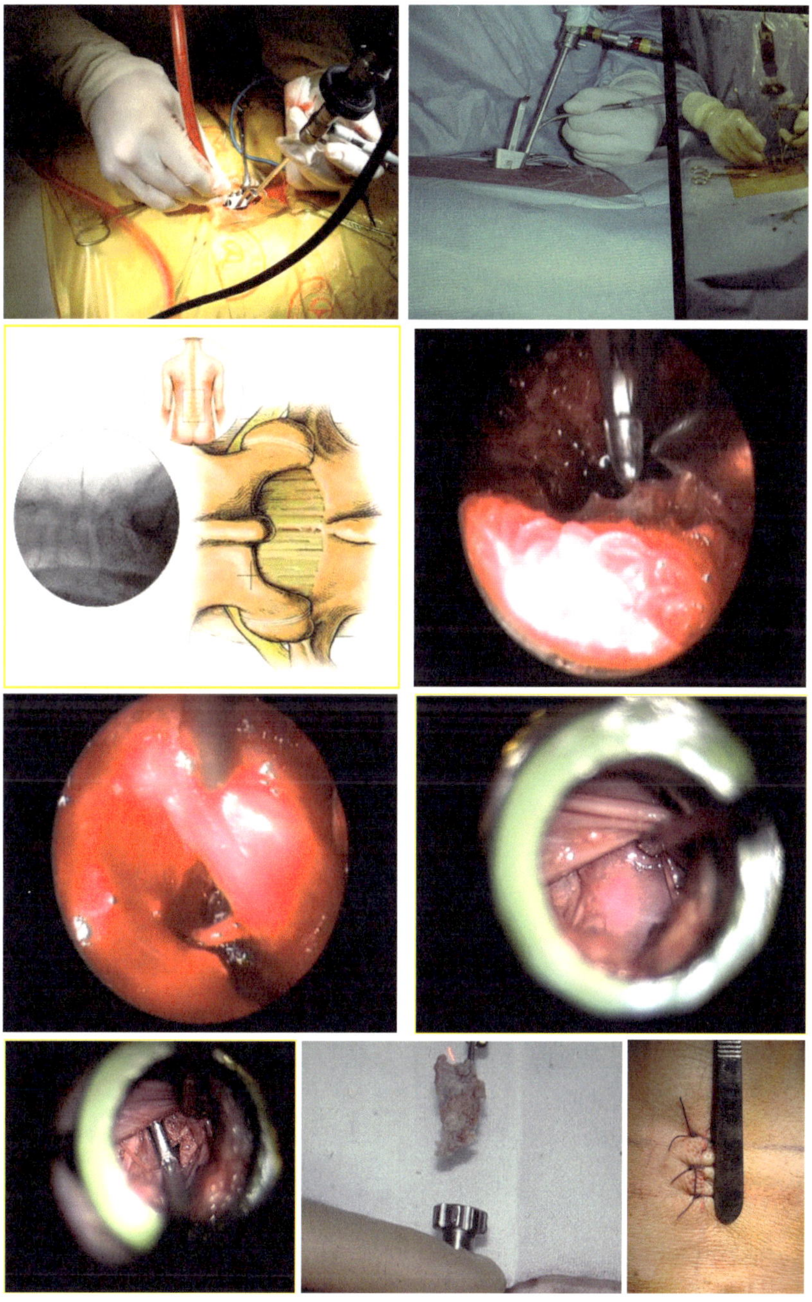

Figure 12. Intraoperative aspects (a-i)

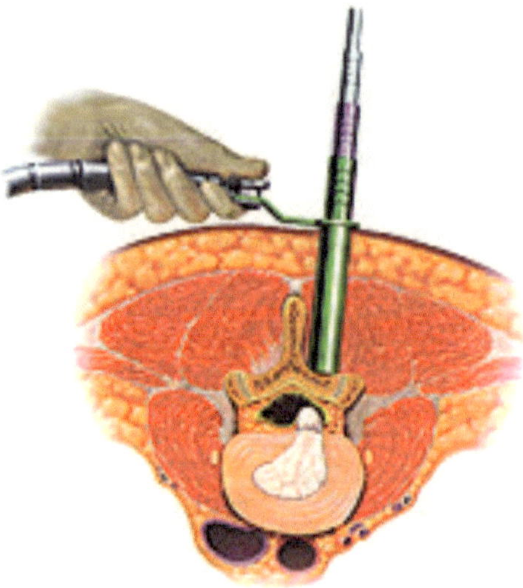

Figure 13. Wolfe & Metronic technique

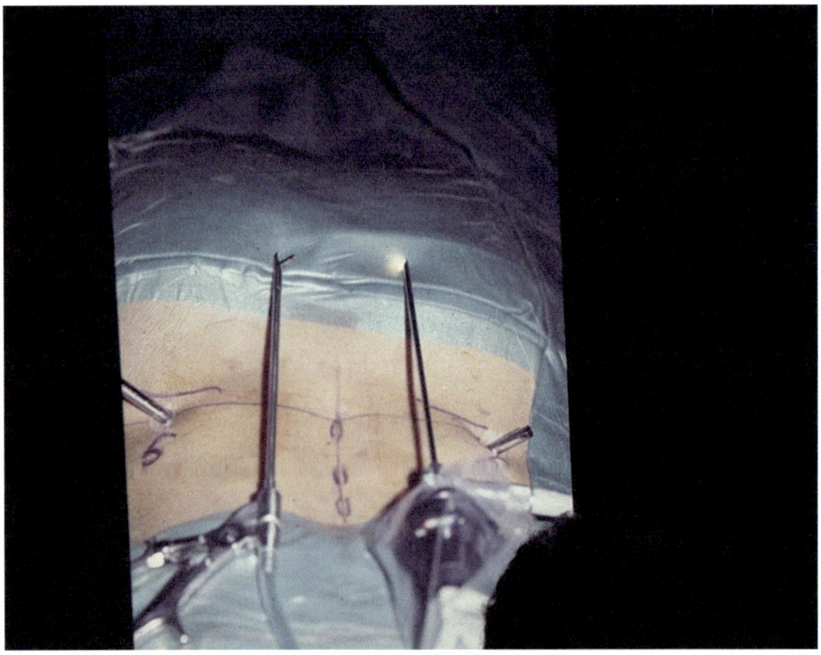

Figure 14. Leu's lateral technique

With endoscopic control intervertebral fusions can be performed either transperithoneal or by thoracoscopy.

http://dx.doi.org/10.5772/54544

5.3. Author's experience and statistical analysis

Between 2006-2011 we had 40 patients with endoscopic discectomy for lumbar disc. 24 males and 16 females, mean age 48 years (35 – 72), lumbar stenosis was associated in 11 cases. Mean follow-up was 15 months.

One patient was reoperated for a fistula of cerebro-spinal fluid, and the defect was sutured using a combined fascial and haemostatic patch. Three patients required revision for a post-operative hematoma or remaining hernia fragment. Hospital stay was in average 3,3 days (2,5). The Waddel score was excellent or good for 91% of patients and Prolo score was excellent or good for 84%. Mean improvement compare with the preoperative status was 65%, as assessed by Oswestry score (Fig.15).

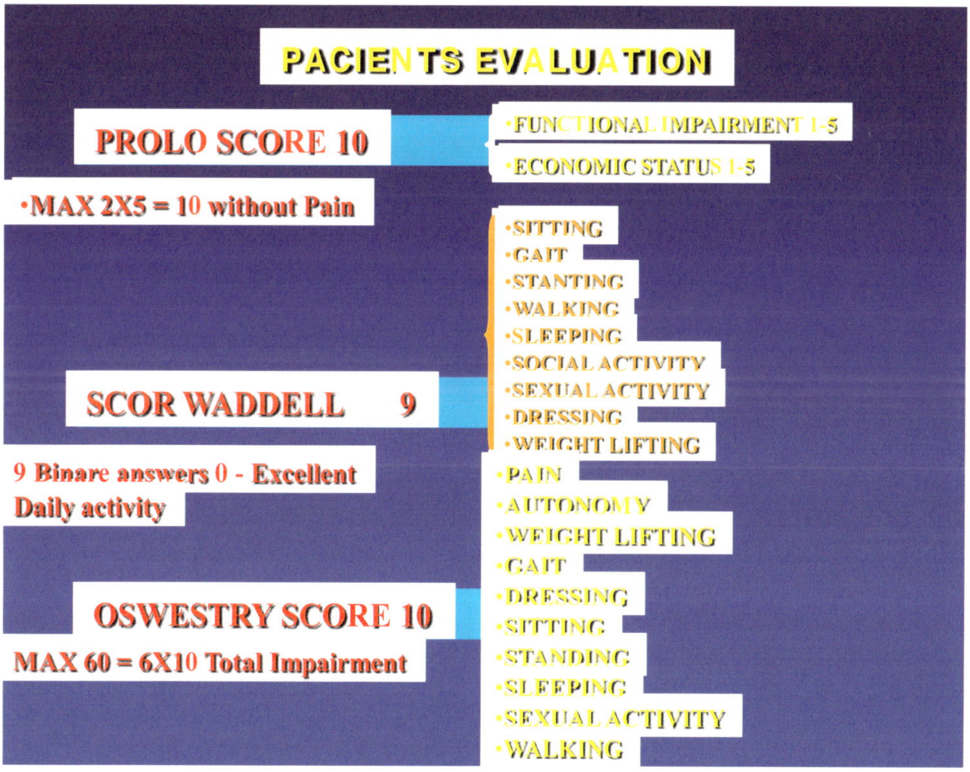

Figure 15. Clinical and Functional evaluation scores

We use anticoagulant therapy for thrombembolism profilaxy. There were no DVT or pulmonary embolism (PE) complications in our series.

We have a type II D anomalous origin nerve roots according to Kadish LJ [8]. About those anomalies, an AOTA Study(1997) on 300 IRM review 20 anomalies (6,7%): 14 conjoint roots, 5 barrel roots and 1 intracanalar anastomosis (Fig.16).

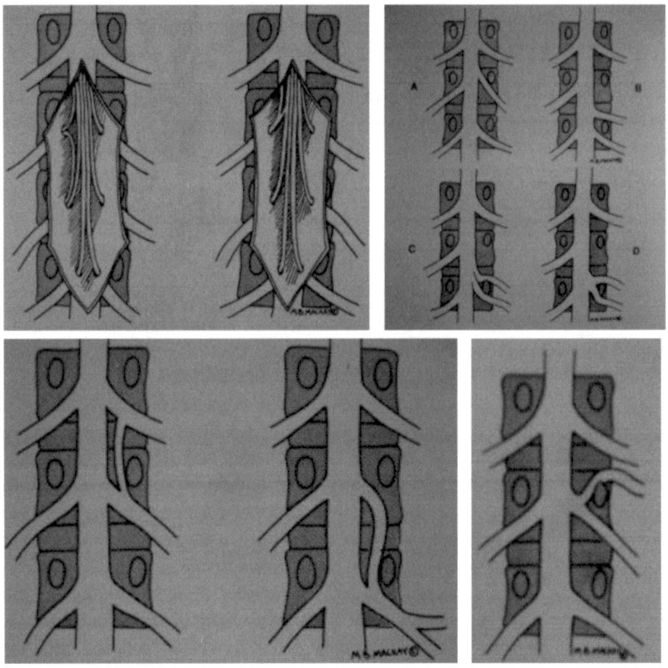

Figure 16. Nerve roots anatomical anomalies [8]

5.4. Postoperative care

5.4.1. Deep venous thrombosis (DVT) prevention

Inspite of minimal surgery, in this spinal surgery DVT is not a rare complication (Weinstein P.R. - 1982).

The use of one of the low-molecular-weight heparins is advisable. One should prolong their use for more than 3 weeks until the complete mobilisation of the pacient.

5.4.2. Mobilisation

In generaly immediate postoperative mobilisation of the patient is achieved. Administration of NSAI is prolonged till 3 days after surgery.

5.4.3. Weight-bearing

In general, walking with weight-bearing is possible after 1 day. Weight lifting is forbited even 1 month postoperatively, in obese patients or those with osteoporotic bone even more.

5.4.4. Complications

The risk of infection is reduced due to: minimal dissection and antibiotics.

Fistula of cerebro-spinal fluid, could be even more frequent comparing to classical surgery, but a revision could be necessary, if the dressing after 2 day is still wet, and fascial patch resolve that. The postoperative hematoma or remaining hernia fragment, are also indications of revision. Nerve roots sectioning or nerve palsy is rare but possible. Mistake of the herniate level, is avoided by floroscopic control.

6. Conclusion

This kind of minimal surgery, by endoscopic herniated disc ablation provide an excellent visualisation, like „ the eye is inside", by a small skin incision, with rapid resumption of activities and a better post-operative comfort.

A bipolar hemostasis could be done.

This surgery is indicated in all stages of herniated lombar disc, with or without canal stenosis.

There is a lower rate of infectious or bleeding complications.

A single dose of antibiotics is admninistrated during surgery and anticoagulant for thrombembolism prophylaxis is done.

Author details

Ştefan Cristea, Florin Groseanu, Andrei Prundeanu, Dinu Gartonea, Andrei Papp, Mihai Gavrila and Dorel Bratu

Clinic of Orthopaedic and Trauma Surgery, St. Pantelimon Hospital, Bucharest, Romania

References

[1] Anthony P.Schnuerer, Julio Gallego, Cristie Manuel – Core Curriculum for Basic Spinal Training – ed. 2009

[2] Antonescu Dinu Mihai, Mihail Buga, Ioan Constantinescu, Nicolae Iliescu – Metode de calcul şi tehnici experimentale de analiza tensiunilor în Biomecanică ed Tehnică Bucureşti 1986

[3] Bar Charts – Quick Study Anatomy Test ed 1998

[4] Bullough P.G. and Boachie-Adjei O. – Atlas of Spinal Diseases – Harcourt Publishers Limited. Ed 1988

[5] Cristea Ştefan, Groseanu F., Prundeanu A. - Caiet De Tehnici Chirurgicale Vol 4 – Tehnici de ortopedie artroscopica ed. medicala Buc 2011 – ISBN 978-973-39-0650-6 si ISBN 978-973-39-0710-7 - pag 257 – 268

[6] Destandau J. "First International Course about Endoscopic Lumbar Microdiscectomy and Lumbar Canal Decompression" 2004 March 25th-26th BORDEAUX

[7] Destandau Jean Microendoscopic surgery DVD 04 2005 ISBN 3-89756-808-X Storz

[8] Kadish L.J., Simmons E.H. - Anomalies of the lumbosacral nerve roots. An anatomical investigation and myelographic study. - J Bone Joint Surg Br. 1984 May;66(3):411-6.

[9] Kieser CW, Jackson R W. Severin Nordentoft: The first arthroscopist. *Arthroscopy* 2001, 17(5):532-5.

[10] Modic MT, Steinberg PM, Ross JS, et al. Degenerative disk disease: Assessment of changes in vertebral body marrow with MR imaging. Radiology 1988;166:193–99

[11] Nigel Palastanga, Derek Field, Roger Soames – Anatomy and Human Movement – Structure and Function, Butterworth – Heinemann Ltd. Oxford ed. – 1990

[12] Watanabe M: History arthroscopic surgery. In Shahriaree H (first edition): O'Connor's Textbook of Arthroscopic surgery. Philadelphia, J.B. Lippincott Co., 1983.

[13] Weinstein P.R. – Anatomy of the lumbar spine . Lumbar Disc Disease – Hardy R.W. ed 1982

Chapter 4

Temporomandibular Joint Arthroscopy *versus* Arthrotomy

Edvitar Leibur, Oksana Jagur and Ülle Voog-Oras

Additional information is available at the end of the chapter

http://dx.doi.org/10.5772/55011

1. Introduction

Although some patients with temporomandibular joint (TMJ) disorders are successfully treated by nonsurgical means or by arthrocentesis or arthroscopic surgery, there is still a group of patients who do not respond to these procedures and for whom an arthrotomy and disc surgery (discoplasty) are necessary. Arthroscopy is an important diagnostic and therapeutic modality in the treatment of TMJ disorders being an alternative to arthrotomy („open" TMJ surgery) and can be very effective in eliminating symptoms as pain, mandibular dysfunction, hypomobility, acute and chronic „closed lock" due to osteoarthritis and arthrosis with adhesive capsulitis, where nonsurgical treatment has been unsuccessful. Bony ankylosis and fibrosis are best managed by open arthrotomy procedures. It has been found that a total of 22 of the 137 arthroscopies were diagnostic only, which resulted in immediate arthrotomy, including arthroplasty, meniscectomy [1]. Arthroscopy is a technique for direct visual inspection of internal joint structures, including biopsy and other surgical procedures performed under visual control. In 1918 Takagi first described arthroscopy of the knee joint examinations using cystoscope [2]. Onishi in 1970 was the first to report arthroscopy of the human temporomandibular joint and the first results were published by him [3,4]. The progress in research and applications of TMJ arthroscopy in joint disease have led to the acceptance of small operative procedures as a safe, minimally invasive means of effectively treating a number of intra-articular and degenerative TMJ problems [5-7]. Arthroscopic surgery has been an effective treatment for TMJ disorders refractory to nonsurgical treatments [8-10]. TMJ arthroscopy has been variously reported as successful in up to 80% of cases where outcome of arthroscopic surgery to the TMJ correlates with the stage of internal derangement [11-13]. Studies have been variable in their scientific methods and some long-term outcomes studies have been completed where both quality of life and functional outcome have been assessed [14-16]. For enabling direct comparison of the clinical results following arthroscopic surgery and open surgery a retrospective study comparing two centers′ results using the Jaw Pain and Function Questionnaire [17] has been performed and these treatment results of open surgery were comparable with arthroscopic treatment results [15].

2. Anatomy of the temporomandibular joint

The temporomandibular joint is the articulation between the mandible and the cranium. The mandibular head (condyle), glenoid (mandibular) fossa, and articular eminence form the TMJ. These joints serve as one anatomic control for both mandibular movement and the occlusion, surrounded by a capsule which consists of fibrous material, and a synovial lining. The capsule is quite thin anteromedially and medially ~ 0,7 mm and thick laterally and posteriorly ~1,8 mm. The inner layer of the capsule or synovial membrane is highly vascularized layer of endothelial origin cells, producing synovial fluid. The capsule stretches from the edge of the mandibular fossa to the neck of the mandible, proximal to the pterygoid fovea, and envelops the articular eminence.Excessive displacement of the mandible is restricted by the joint capsule and ligaments. Nearist to the joint is temporomandibular joint ligament, which consists of a fibrous thickening in the lateral joint capsule. This ligament extends from the inferior surface of the posterior aspect of the zygomatic arch to the lateral part of the neck of the condyle. It functions by preventing lateral dislocation and it also prevents medial dislocation (Figure 1a). The two other ligaments are described in conventional anatomical descriptions of the joint, although it is doubtful whether either has a functional role. The sphenomandibular ligament running from the lingula shielding the opening of the inferior alveolar canal to the spine of the sphenoid. This ligament represents the residual perichondrium of Meckel's cartilage. The second ligament is the stylomandibular ligament running from the spine of the sphenoid to the angle of the mandible and represent the free border of the deep cervical fascia (Figure 1b).

The articular surface of the mandible is the upper and anterior surface of the condyle, lined by dense, avascular, fibrous connective tissue. A layer of hyaline cartilage covers the articulating cortical bone. The adult human condyle is about 15 to 20 mm from side to side and 8 to 10 mm from front to back. The articular surface is convex when viewed from the side and less when viewed from the front. Glenoid fossa is the concavity within the temporal bone. The anterior wall is formed by the articular eminence of the temporal bone and its posterior wall by the tympanic plate, which also forms the anterior wall of the external auditory meatus. An articular disc is interposed between the temporal bone and the mandible, dividing the articular space into upper and lower compartments (Figure 2).

The interposed fibrocartilaginous disc has a bow-tie-shaped biconcave morphology. The anterior and posterior ridges of the disc are termed anterior and posterior bands and are longer in the mediolateral than in the anteroposterior dimension. The smaller anterior band attaches to the articular eminence, condylar head, and joint capsule. The posterior band blends with highly vascularized, loose connective tissue, the bilaminar zone, and the capsule, the bilaminar zone residing in the retrodiscal space in the mandibular fossa and attaching to the condyle and temporal bone. Medially and laterally, the disc is firmly attached to the capsule and the

http://dx.doi.org/10.5772/55011

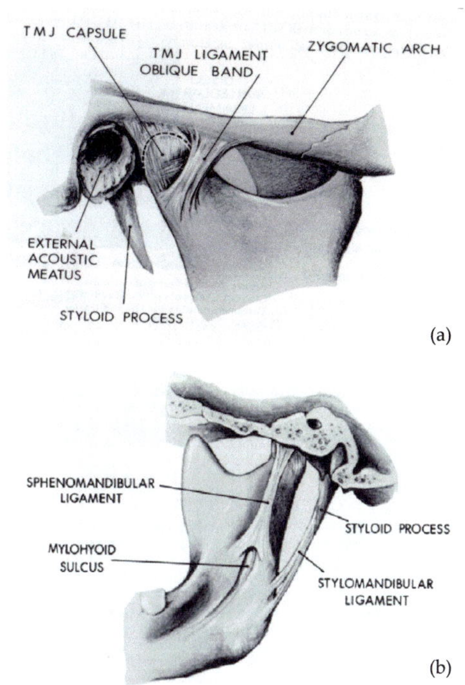

Figure 1. a. The temporomandibular ligament by M. M. Ash (In:Wheeler´s dental anatomy, physiology and occlusion, W.B. Saunders Company, Philadelphia 1993). b. The sphenomandibular and stylomandibular ligaments by M. M. Ash (In: Wheeler´s dental anatomy, physiology and occlusion, W.B. Saunders Company, Philadelphia 1993).

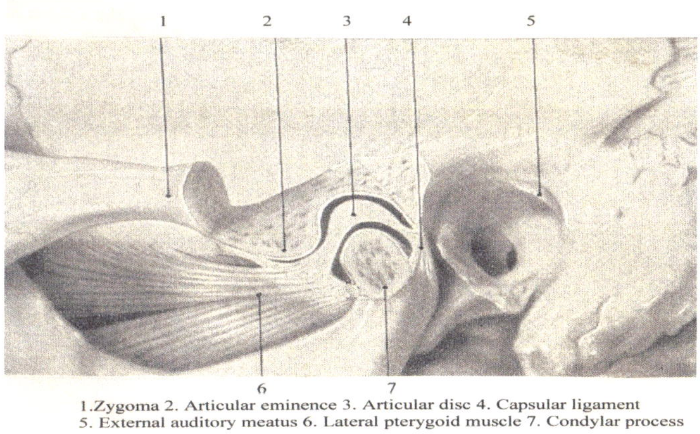

Figure 2. A sagittal section through the left temporomandibular joint.

condylar neck. Anteromedially, it is attached to the superior part of the pterygoid muscle. In a physiologic joint, the disc is positioned between the mandibular head inferiorly and the articular eminence anteriorly and superiorly when the jaw is closed. The posterior band of the disc lies within 10° of the 12 o'clock position. The medial and lateral corners of the disc align with the condylar borders and do not bulge laterally or medially. When the jaw is opened, the disc slides into a position between the mandibular head and articular eminence. The loose tissue of the bilaminar zone allows the remarkable range of motion of the disc. The attachments of the disc prevent luxation during opening. A triangular lateral ligament acts as a strong lateral stabilizer and inhibits the posterior translation of the mandibular head. The muscles of mastication are responsible for the complex movement of the jaw. The temporal, medial pterygoid, and masseter muscles facilitate jaw closure. Mouth opening is effected by coordinated action of the lateral pterygoid, mylohyoid, digastric, and suprahyoid muscles. The lateral pterygoid muscle and part of the fibers of the masseter and medial pterygoid muscles effect the anterior translation of the mandible. The superior belly of the lateral pterygoid muscle originates from the greater sphenoid wing and inserts on the disc. Subsequently, the superior belly plays a key role in upholding the physiologic position of the disc as it pulls the disc forward when the jaw is opened, in a combined translation and rotation. The inferior head of the lateral pterygoid muscle stretches from the lateral lamina of the pterygoid process to the pterygoid fovea. The medial pterygoid muscle originates from the pterygoid fossa and inserts near the medial aspect of the mandibular angle [18].The blood supply to the TMJ, outer and inner ear is provided mainly by branches from an internal maxillary artery as follows: temporal superficial artery, superior auricular artery, anterior tympanic artery and pterygoid artery. Innervation is provided by the auriculotemporal nerve (sensory branch of the mandibular nerve), deep temporal nerve, masseteric nerve. Sensory cervical sympathetic ramifications are going to disc and capsule.The auriculotemporal nerve runs medial to the joint, then runs laterally, crossing the condylar neck, where it divides into branches to innervate the capsule, disc attachments, the tympanic membrane, the anterior surface of the cochlea, the upper part of the auricule, the tragus of the ear, the skin lining, the external auditory meatus, the temporal region (Figure 3) [19].

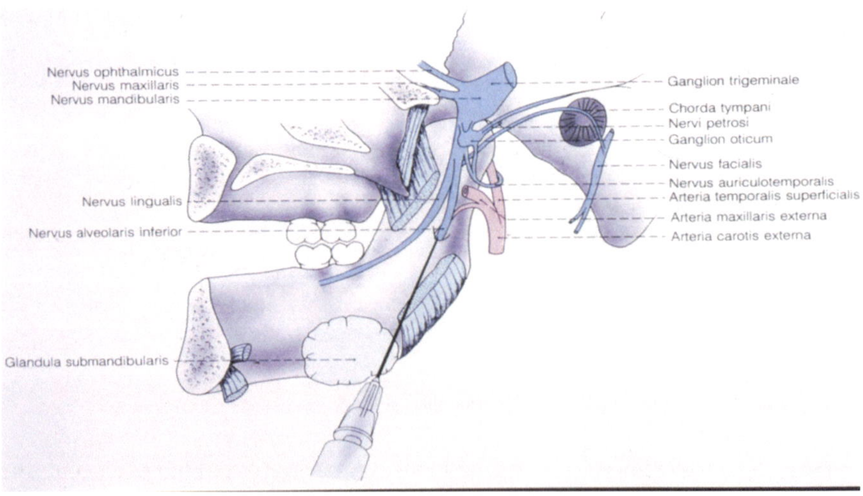

Figure 3. Branches of trigeminal nerve. Innervation and blood supply of temporomandibular joint (by R. Schmelzle, 1989).

http://dx.doi.org/10.5772/55011

Nerve receptors as Ruffin receptors, Golgi tendon organs, Vater-Pacini corpuscules free nerve endings are in the capsule and substance P nerve fibres are also available in both the auriculotemporal and masseteric nerves, and have been demonstrated in the capsule, disc attachments but they are not present in the disc. The Vater-Pacini corpuscules are large "onion-like" encapsulated pressure receptors. The surrounding concentric lamellae respond to distortion and generate an action potential in the unmyelinated fiber in the core (Figure 4).

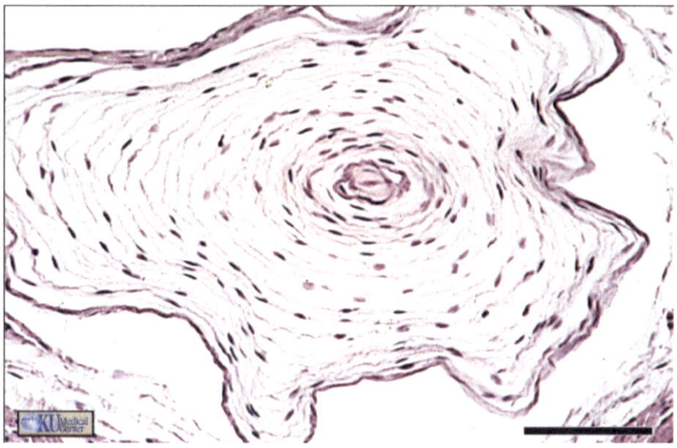

Figure 4. The Vater-Pacini corpuscule. (http://www.kumc.edu/instruction/medicine/anatomy/histoweb/nervous.htm)

3. Classification of TMJ disorders

1. Inflammatory arthritis:
   - acute, chronic
   - infectious: nonspecific, specific (gonococcal, syphilitic, tuberculous, Lyme disease associated arthritis)
2. Osteoarthritis/arthrosis (most often disorder)
3. Injuries:
   - macrotrauma as luxations, concussion, fracture
   - multiple instances of microtrauma
4. Ankylosis (fibrous, fibro-osseous, osseous)
5. Systemic conditions affecting the TMJ: rheumatoid arthritis, juvenile arthritis, psoriatric arthritis, Sjögren syndrome, ankylosing spondylitis (namely seropositive), scleroderma, mixed connective tissue disease, gout, pseudogout, calcium pyrophosphate deposition disease (CPDD)

6. Tumours (benign and malignant)

7. Congenital disturbances: I & II branchial arch malformations, condylar hypo-, hyperplasia, idiopathic condylar resorption.

4. Aetiology and pathogenesis of temporomandibular joint disorders

4.1. Aetiology

Main aetiological factors of TMJ disorders are as follows: systemic diseases (rheumatoid arthritis, psoriasis, pseudogout, ankylosing spondylitis etc.), secondary inflammatory component from the neighbouring regions (otitis, maxillary sinusitis, tonsillitis), trauma (chronical), prevalence of dental arch defects *e.g.* missing of molar teeth [20], malocclusion, endocrinological disturbances, odontogenic infections (third molars). Osteoarthritis is an inflammatory process, being most frequent TMJ disorder [6]. In systemic diseases (rheumatoid arthritis, psoriasis etc.) involvement of TMJ occurs [21]. Osteoarthritis refers to an inflammatory condition affecting the bony strructures of the joint that results in destructive changes of hard tissues, and the presence of fibrillations, adhesions. The condition referred to as osteoarthrosis represents a subacute or chronic process that has inflammatory components (inflammatory mediators and markers), identified in the synovial fluid and tissues [22].

Presence of specific bacterial species in the synovial fluid have been found [23]. Serum antibodies against *Chlamydia spp.* in patients with monoarthritis of the TMJ have been occurred. An association may exist between the presence of *Chlamydia trachomatis* and TMJ disease [24].

4.2. Pathogenesis

Knowledge about the pathogenesis on a molecular level of disorders of the TMJ has been improved in recent years giving a possibility to use these data for the evidence based treatment. Inflammation mainly affects the posterior disc attachement [6,10]. Several inflammatory mediators play an important role in the pathogenesis of TMJ diseases as tumor necrosis factor α (TNFα), interleukin-1β (IL-1β), prostaglandin E_2 (PGE_2), leukotrien B_4 (LkB_4), matrix metalloproteinases (MMP_s), serotonin- 5-hydroxytryptamine (5-HT) [22,25]. MMP-s are responsible for the metabolism of extracellular matrix, being an early marker to determine TMJ arthritis. High level of MMP-3 has been determined in the synovial fluid in TMJ osteoarthritis patients [26]. Serotonin, mediator of pain and inflammation, is produced in the enterocromaffin cells of the gastrointestinal mucosa and absorbed by platelets. It is produced also in the synovial membrane and is present in the synovial fluid and in blood in case of rheumatoid arthritis and is involved in the mediation of TMJ pain in systemic inflammatory joint diseases [27,28]. It plays a role also in bone metabolism [29]. Tissue response in case of inflammation is as follows: vasodilatation, extravasation, releasing of mediators, activation of nociceptors, release of neuropeptides as substance P (SP), neuropeptide Y (NPY), which stimulate releasing of histamin and serotonin from afferent nerve endings and hyperalgesia in TMJ occurs.

http://dx.doi.org/10.5772/55011

5. Diagnostics of the temporomandibular joint disorders

5.1. Clinical data

The most frequent complaint is pain, joint sounds and a decrease in the maximal interincisal opening (MIO), which normal values are between 35 -50 mm. Mouth opening is recorded by asking the patient to open maximally, and the distance between maxillary and mandibular incisors tip is measured (Figure 5). Locking and deviation of mandible is recorded as present or absent.

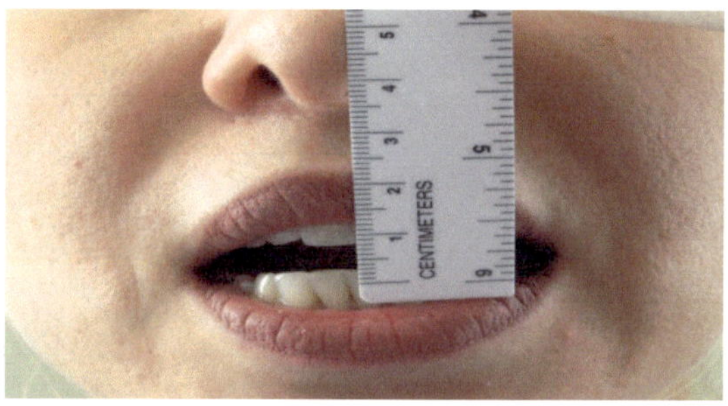

Figure 5. Female patient 22 yrs. with difficulty in opening the mouth, maximal interincisal opening (MIO) is only 6 mm.

The following symptoms as pain (at rest, during maksimum mouth opening and upon chewing), tenderness to digital palpation of the joint, sounds (clicking, crepitation), restricted mandibular mobility *e.g.* difficulty in opening the mouth, intermittent lock, closed lock, stiffness in the morning are observed. Visual analog scales (VAS) are very useful instruments to estimate the intensity of the pain or the level of suffering that patient has been experiencing. The stages of disease are usually classified according to Wilkes [30], (Table 1) by reviewing the case histories, clinical data, radiological records (computerized tomography images incl. cone beam computer tomography), magnetic resonance images, orthopantomography and/or plain radiographs by Schüller, Parma.

Symptom related factors obtained by questionnaire, the scores pre- and posttreatment MIO and VAS for pain are to be documentated and compared. Joint pain is assessed with 100mm visual analogue scale with end points marked „no pain" and „worst pain ever experienced". The absence of pain is scored as 0. If pain is present the patient is asked to select marked field from 1mm to 100 mm. It is known that inflammation often is accompanied by pain. Evaluation and estimation of the impact of pain is a complicated matter, since pain has many different ways to interfere with everyday life. The impact of pain on the health status and quality of life in patients with chronic inflammatory joint diseases has been recognized, but there is a lack of knowledge about the specific impact of TMJ pain on daily activities in patients with clinical involvement of the TMJ. A scale for measuring the activity of daily living (ADL) [31] of patients with TMJ disorders for assessment of the restriction of activities is a useful tool [14,16,32].

I.Early stage
A. Clinical: No significant mechanical symptoms other than opening reciprocal clicking; no pain or limitation of motion
B. Radiologic: Slight forward displacement, good anatomic contour of the disc, negative tomograms, no bone structure changes
C. Pathoanatomy: Excellent anatomic form; slight anterior displacement, passive in-coordination demonstrable
II. Early intermediate stage
A. Clinical: One or more episodes of pain: beginning major mechanical problems consisting of mid-to-late opening loud clicking; transient catching and locking
B. Radiologic: Slight forward displacement; beginning disc deformity, slight thickening of posterior edge; negative tomograms, no bone structure changes
C. Pathoanatomy: Anterior disk displacement; early disk deformity; good central articulating area
III. Intermediate stage
A. Clinical: Multiple episodes of pain; major mechanical symptoms consisting of locking (intermittent or fully closed): restriction of motion, function difficulties
B. Radiologic: Anterior disc displacement with significant deformity or prolapse of disc (increased thickening of posterior edge), negative tomograms, no bone structure changes
C. Pathoanatomy: Marked anatomic disc deformity with anterior displacement; no hard tissue changes
IV. Late intermediate stage
A. Clinical: Slight increase in severity over intermediate stage
B. Radiologic: Increase in severity over intermediate stage; positive tomograms showing early-to-moderate degenerative changes - flattening of eminence, deformation of condylar head, erosions, sclerosis
C. Pathoanatomy: Increase in severity over intermediate stage; hard tissue degenerative remodelling of both bearing surfaces (osteophytes), multiple adhesions in anterior and posterior recesses; no perforation of disc or attachments
V. Late stage
A. Clinical: Characterized by crepitus, variable and episodic pain, chronic restriction of motion and difficulty with function
B. Radiologic: Disc or attachment perforation, filling defects, gross anatomic deformity of disk and hard tissues, positive tomograms with essentially degenerative arthritic changes
C. Pathoanatomy: Degenerative changes of disc and hard tissues, perforation of posterior attachement, multiple adhesions, osteophytes, flattening of condyle and eminence, subcortical cyst formation

Table 1. Classification for internal derangement of the TMJ by Wilkes (1989).

5.2. Radiographic investigations

Radiographic changes of the TMJ are evaluated by orthopantomography (OPTG), computed tomography (CT), magnet resonance imaging (MRI) [8,21,22,33] as well as ultrasonography [34]. OPTG is mainly used to demonstrate the structural bone changes in the TMJ and it has the advantage of being easily available but gives limited information about the above mentioned joint. By evaluating the OPTGs the following radiographic signs of bone structural changes can be achieved such as presence of erosions, flattening and osteophytes of the condyle as well as of the temporal bone [35]. Erosion in condyles in the radiographs is scored as follows: score 1 - very slight erosion; score 2 - erosion on top of the condyle; score 3 - half of condyle is eroded; score 4 - condyle totally eroded [36]. The first report of TMJ CT was published by Suarez et al. [37] and this method is superior to plain transcranial or transmaxillary imaging for detecting bone changes. CT allows detailed three-dimensional examination of the TMJ and it is capable to detect even small bone changes not demonstrable by conventional tomographic procedures [38, 39]. The CT sections are evaluated for presence of radiographic signs of bone changes within three regions (lateral, central and medial) of the mandibular and temporal part (eminence) of the TMJ. The recording of the signs is made in the axial, coronal and sagittal views [22, 40]. The changes are defined as follows: erosion - a local area with decreased density of the cortical joint surface including or not including adjacent subcortical bone (Figure 6), sclerosis - a local area with increased density of the cortical bony joint surface that may extend into the subcortical bone (Figure 7), subchondral pseudocyst - a well defined, local area of bone rarefication underneath, an intact cortical outlining of the joint surface, flattening – a flat bony contour deviating from the convex form (Figure 8). The grade of the total changes of the TMJ can be evaluated according to the scoring system [41]. Not treated properly and immediately a juvenile trauma to the TMJ area can lead to ankylosis (Figure 9). 3-D reconstruction of the mandible gives a possibility to find the fracture of the condyle not diagnosed in time (Figure 10).

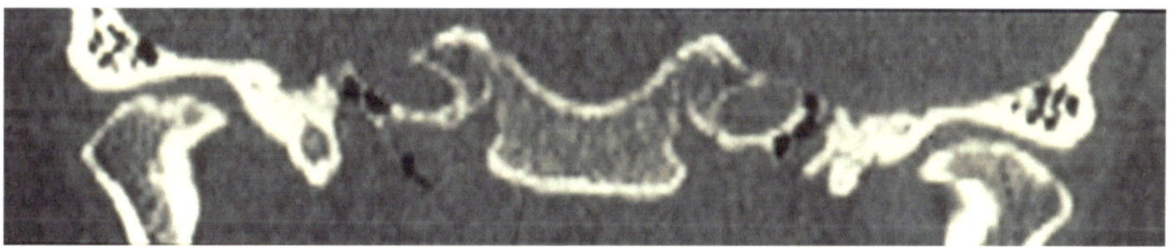

Figure 6. Osteoarthritis of the TMJ, signs of erosions on the surfaces of the condyles in a coronal view of the CT.

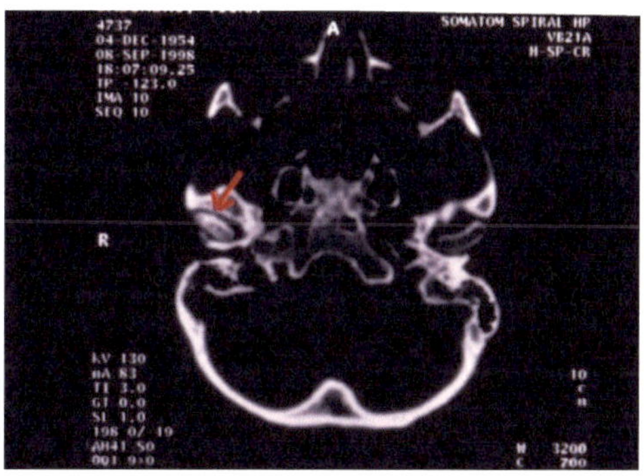

Figure 7. Axial view of the CT from the head, sign of sclerosis in the medial and central parts of the right condyle of the mandible (red arrow).

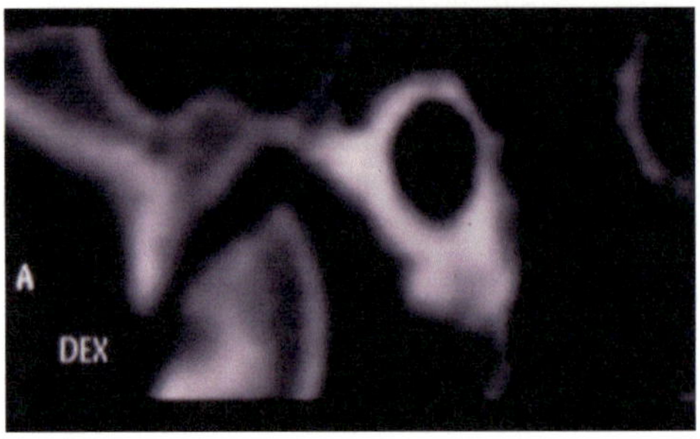

Figure 8. Sagittal view of the CT from the temporomandibular joint, sign of flattening of the left mandibular condyle.

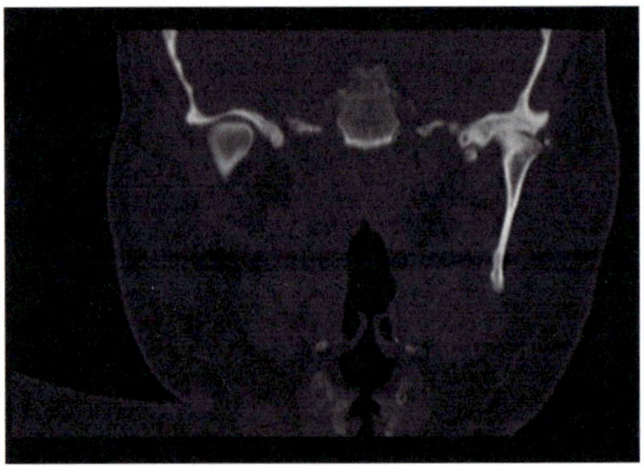

Figure 9. Coronal view of the the CT, osseous ankylosis of the left TMJ.

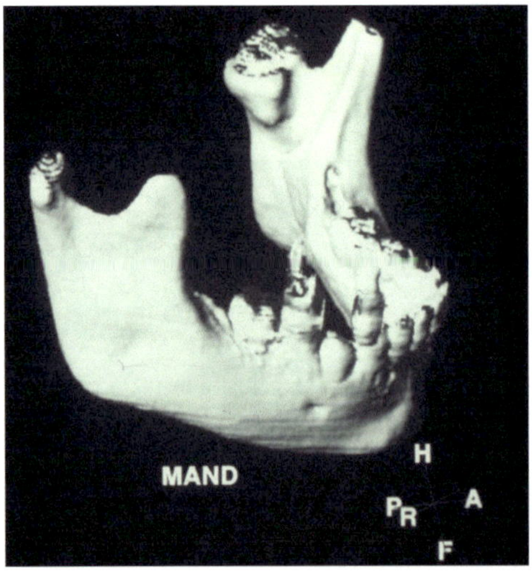

Figure 10. Male patient 9 yrs, trauma has been ~ 5 years ago, fracture of the left condyle is evident, displaced medially.

http://dx.doi.org/10.5772/55011

Foreign bodies in case of calcium pyrophosphate deposition disease (CPPD) crystals and synovial chondromatosis granules may by diagnosed radiographically (Figure 11, 12).

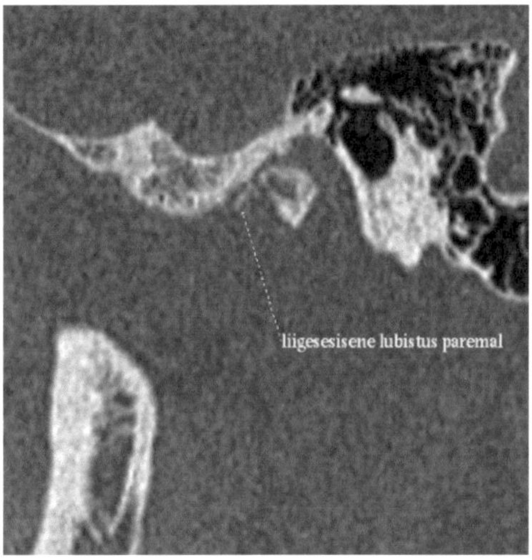

Figure 11. Sagittal view of the CT, left TMJ in an open mouth position, the calcifications in the joint space are found.

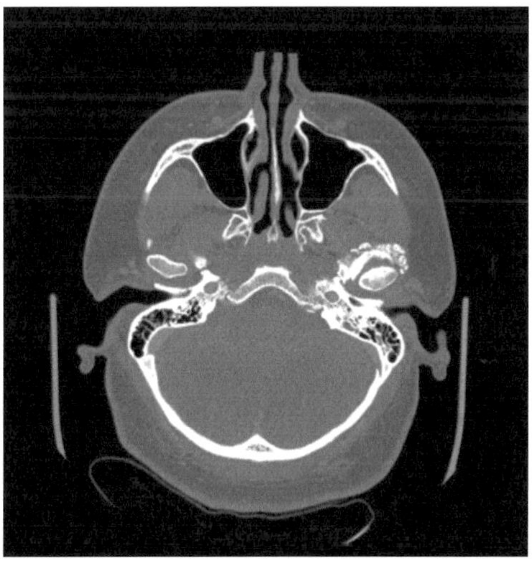

Figure 12. Axial view of the CT, granules of synovial chondromatosis are in the left TMJ.

MRI has diagnostic value for internal derangements of the TMJ and rapidly surpassing CT as the imaging method of choice (Figure 13, 14). Sections in the oblique sagittal plane (*i.e.* perpendicular to the horizontal long axis of the mandibular condyle) and oblique coronal plane (*i.e.* parallel with the long axis of the condyle), and bilateral temporomandibular base surface coils are used for obtaining the image [39]. Disc displacement without reduction is found by using MRI in at least one of the joints in 75% of the subjects and in 54% of all the joints imaged.

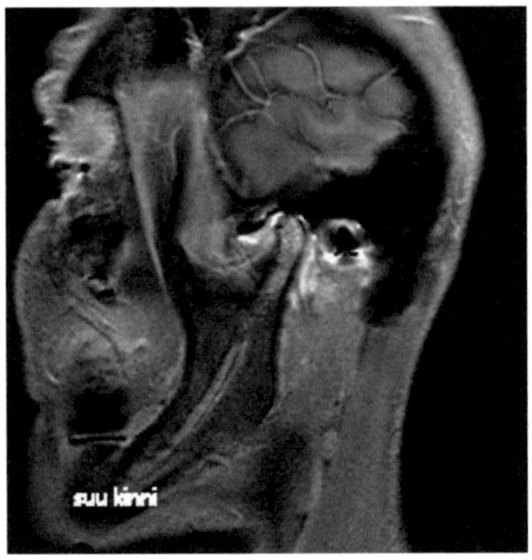

Figure 13. Sagittal view of the MRI in the closed mouth position in a patient with internalderangement of the left TMJ. Anterior disc displacement, hypoplastic condyle, destruction of the disc. Changes of bone structures, effusion in the anterior recess.

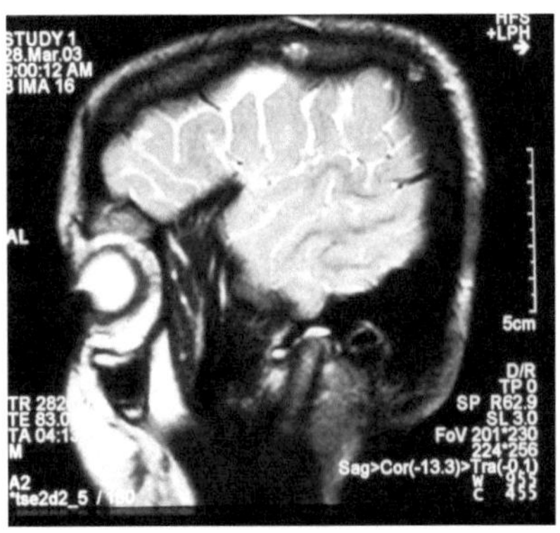

Figure 14. Sagittal view of the MRI in a patient with internal derangement of the left TMJ. Anterior disc displacement, destruction of the disc. Changes in the bone structures, effusion in the anterior recess.

The biting device (MEDRAD; Pittsburg) which enables dynamic imaging can be used as bite blocks during the open jaw phase of the imaging procedure [42]. Ultrasonography has been a helpful diagnostic approach for patients with TMJ disorders, having a possibility to diagnose with considerable reliability when compared with MRI and being a sensitive tool for assessing joint function [43].

6. Temporomandibular joint arthroscopy

6.1. Indications for TMJ arthroscopy

The treatment decision must be based on a patient examination evaluation that integrates the imaging and clinical findings, including the history and the other diagnostic data.

Indications for arthroscopy are radiological bone changes in TMJ characteristic to osteoarthritis with disc displacement or deformity and non effectiveness of conservative treatment with NSAIDs, intraoral splints or arthrocentesis. Arthroscopic surgery has been used to treat anteriorly displaced, nonreducing discs. Various techniques have been used as: lysis of adhesions and joint lavage, anterior disc release, lateral capsular release, scarification of the retrodiscal region with a laser. Arthroscopic electrothermal capsulorrhaphy is performed using a standard double puncture operative arthroscopy with a Hol: YAG laser [44]. In practice, the decision to operate and the choice of the method seems to be a matter of the individual surgeon´s training, experience, and attitude toward the surgical management of TMJ disorders. Involvement of the TMJ in patients with rheumatoid arthritis or other connective tissue diseases is rather common and arthroscopy with simultaneous biopsy is indicated in these situations. Posttraumatic complaints may also be an indication for arthroscopy. Arthroscopy is contraindicated in case of acute arthritis. In these situations as large medial osteophytes on the condyle, large central cartilaginous perforations, fibrous, fibro-osseous, osseous ankylosis are better to handle *via* open reduction. Arthocentesis is considered as an interventing treatment modality between nonsurgical treatment and arthroscopic surgery. All cases for arthroscopy are usually classified as advanced Wilkes [30] stages IV and V, in rare cases stage III (Table 1).

6.2. Prearthroscopic procedures

Temporomandibular arthroscopy is usually done on an outpatient basis in the hospital. If diagnostic arthroscopy is followed by arthrotomy, the patient is admitted for postoperative care. Arthroscopy is performed under general anaesthesia with nasotracheal intubation which makes possible to manipulate the mandible during the operation. Both the surgeon and the assistant surgeon should have direct visibility of the monitor. First the zygomatic arch and the condyle are palpated. The condyle is then forced in anterior position by the assistant and the preauricular concavity is formed in the skin, marking a point for the injection. Although various arthroscopic approaches to the TMJ have been described, the one most commonly used is the posterolateral approach to the upper joint space. After the condylar head of the TMJ has been determined, a marking line and puncture points are made on the skin surface (Figure 15).

The puncture site is located by manipulating the mandible anterio-inferiorly. For distension of the superior compartement and in order to avoid iatrogenic damage to the cartilaginous surfaces during introduction of the trocar, 0,5 – 1,0 % lidocain solution 2,0 mL with 1: 200 000 epinephrine is inserted to distend the superior compartment dilatation of capsule, in order to get hemostasis and postoperative analgesia. The solution is injected with a 27-gauge needle, which is aimed in a medial and slightly anterio-superior direction until the contact with the

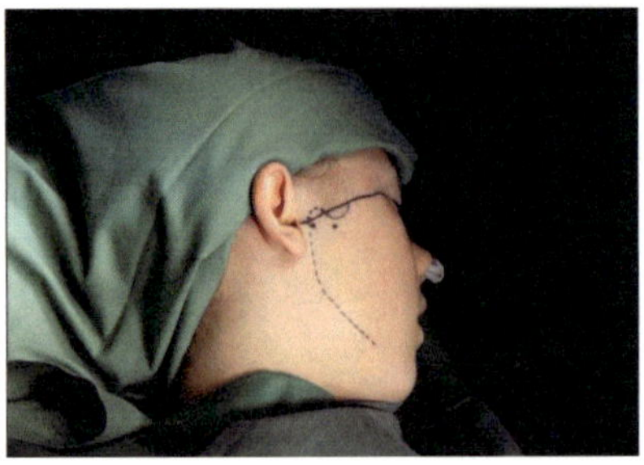

Figure 15. A marking line and the puncture points on the skin surface for TMJ arthroscopy.

glenoid fossa is achieved. The posterior recess of the superior joint space is reached when there is a backflow into the syringe of the solution injected into the joint space (Figure 16).

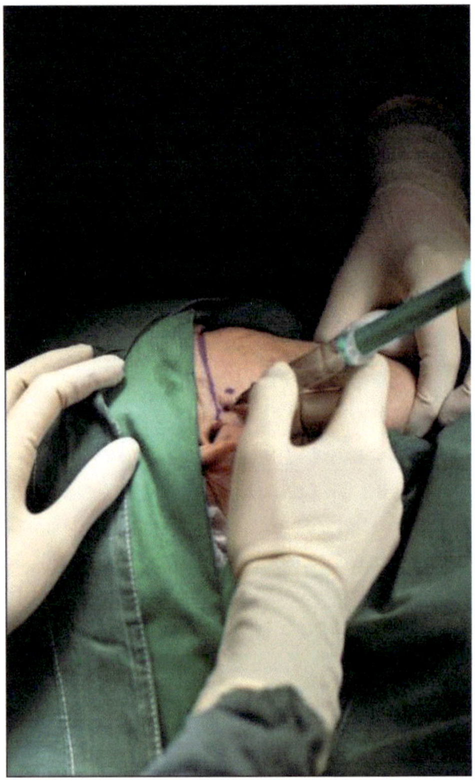

Figure 16. Distension of the superior compartment with 2% lidocaine solution.

6.3. Technique for arthroscopy

Usually arthroscope KARL STORZ GmbH & Co.KG is used. Overall view of the set is given in the Figure 17.

http://dx.doi.org/10.5772/55011

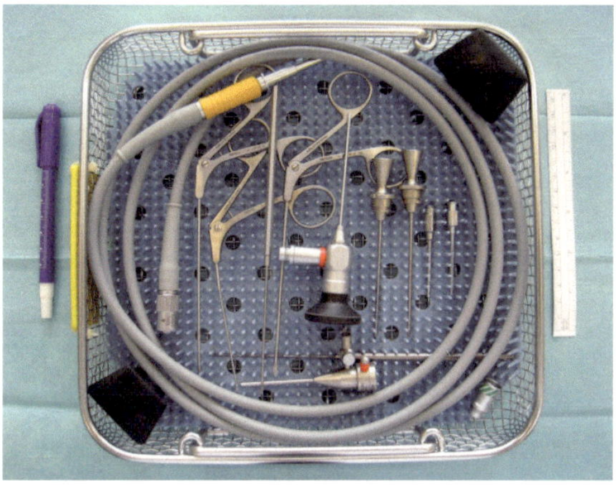

Figure 17. Overall view of the instruments set of arthroscope KARL STORZ GmbH & Co.KG with forward oblique - telescope 30° (HOPKINS®).

Through the small skin incision 0,75 – 1,0 cm from the center of the *tragus* at the injection site the lateral capsule is punctured with a sharp trocar in an arthroscopic sheath inserted in the same direction as the previous injection needle. The sharp trocar is exchanged for a blunt one and the arhroscopic sheath is advanced further into the upper joint space. Puncture with arthroscope sheath (trocar) with a blunt obturator inserted into upper posterior recess is performed angling it medially upward ~ 2,5 cm. Another skin incision is made ~ 0,75 cm from the first skin incision in anterolateral direction for outflow cannula to be inserted into the upper joint anterior recess. Following insertion of the trocar (diameter 1,8 mm, length 4 cm) into the joint space, blunt obturator is removed and forward-oblique telescope 30º (HOPKINS®), diameter 1,9 mm, length 6,5 cm, fiber optic light transmission incorporated is inserted (Figure 18). The inferior joint space is seldom entered because of the limited area makes it difficult to insert the trocar.

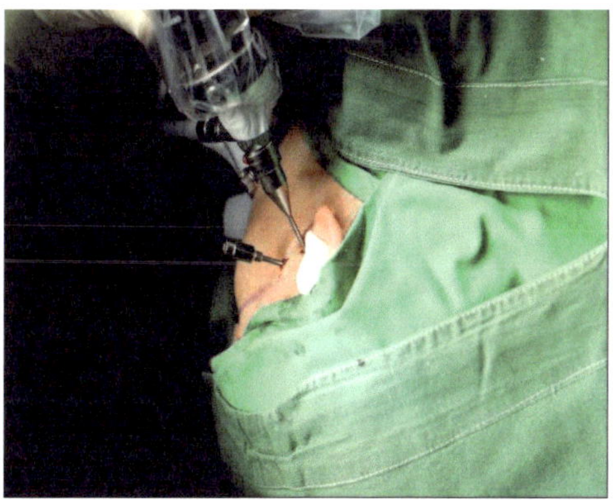

Figure 18. Forward-oblique telescope 30° (HOPKINS®) fiber optic light transmission incorporated and outflow cannula are inserted into the upper joint space.

Initial recognition of anatomical structures as the superior surface of the disc, articular fossa, and internal aspects of the posterior and medial capsule is performed. The fluid level in the arthroscope sheath should move with the jaw, confirming that the sheath is correctly positioned in the joint upper space. The upper joint compartment is examined from the posterior pouch *via* the intermediate zone to the anterior pouch. Disc may give the impression of being obstructed against the arthrotic surface of the temporal cartilage. The anterior part of the disc surface looks usually smooth and collagen fibres could clearly seen. The condylar cartilage is normally smooth, but in case of pathology *e.g.* in osteoarthritis where irregularities of the surface as erosions, osteophyts can be seen. Sever arthrotic changes of both fossa cartilage and disc may also observed. Adhesions between the disc and glenoid fossa are quite common. In rare cases the arthrotic or inflammatory changes are found in the anterior recess. Upper compartment is swept clear under constant irrigation with isotonic saline solution. This manipulation allow translation of the disc along the eminence, allowing the condyle to complete its natural path. After the diagnostic arthroscopy has been completed, either forceps, palpation hook or blunt probe are used to cut fibres, mainly fibers of the pterygoid muscle anterior to the disc, in order to reduce pull in the anterior direction and facilitate repositioning of the disc. Cutting of adhesions facilitate repositioning of the disc. During arthroscopy a sweeping procedure between the disc and fossa released the adhesions and fibrillations increasing the mobility in the joint. Release of the adhesions and fibrillations of the superior suface of the disc and shaving the surface of articular fossa in the upper joint compartment are performed with the aid of a blunt obturator or hook and with grasping forceps, scissors or double-edged knife. Removal of the superficial layer of cortical bone induces capillar bleeding stimulating formation of fibrocartilage on bone. Quite often a displaced disc may be found during arthroscopy. Surgical procedure is completed by irrigating the joint space to remove small tissue fragments. The outflowing fluid is collected and may be retained for diagnostic purposes. Arthroscopic lysis and lavage includes also a lateral release of the upper joint compartment performed with the aid of the blunt obturator or hook. Thus the locked disc could be mobilized sufficiently.

6.4. Analysis of arthroscopic findings

Clinical, radiographic and arthroscopic findings in patients who underwent arthroscopy are given in Table 2 [10].

Arthroscopic findings are as follows: irregularities of joint surfaces, foldings and synovitis – hyperaemia of the inner wall, localising also in the posterior part of the disc, intra-articular fibrous adhesions, intracapsular adhesions, fibrillations of superior surface of the disc and arthrotic lesions of temporal cartilage, pseudowalls, foreign bodies - chondromatosis (Figure 19, 20, 21, 22a, 22b, 23).

Signs and symptoms	**Sum**	**% abn**	**Radiographic findings**	**Sum**	**% abn**	**Arthroscopic findings**	**Sum**	**% abn**
Pain	25	86	Flattening	10	34	Adhesions	29	100
Hypomobility	23	79	Bone cyst / Subchondral pseudocycts	9	31	Chondromatosis	**5**	**17**
Closed lock	5	17	Erosions	20	69	Fibrillations	22	**76**
Intermittent lock	5	17	Reduced space	10	34	Synovitis	**9**	**31**
Deviation	4	14	Sclerosis	8	27	Eburneation of fossa	15	**52**
			Hypomobility of condyle	4	14	Displaced disc	**23**	**23**
			Osteophyts	5	17			

Sum = total number of patients with findings; % abn = percentage of individuals with abnormal findings.

Table 2. Clinical, radiographic and arthroscopic findings in patients who underwent arthroscopy (N=29).

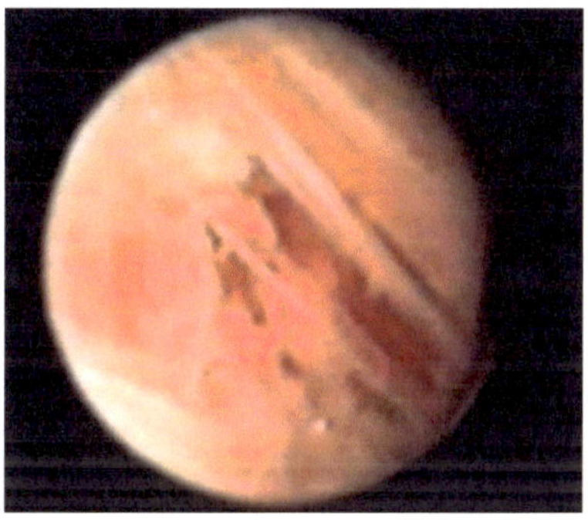

Figure 19. Posterior recess of the superior compartment of the right TMJ. Fibrillations and pronounced adhesions with appearance irregularities of condylar surface, hyperaemia in the posterior capsular wall. Synovial chondromatosis granule is in the 6 o´clock position. A greater amount of floating debris is noted.

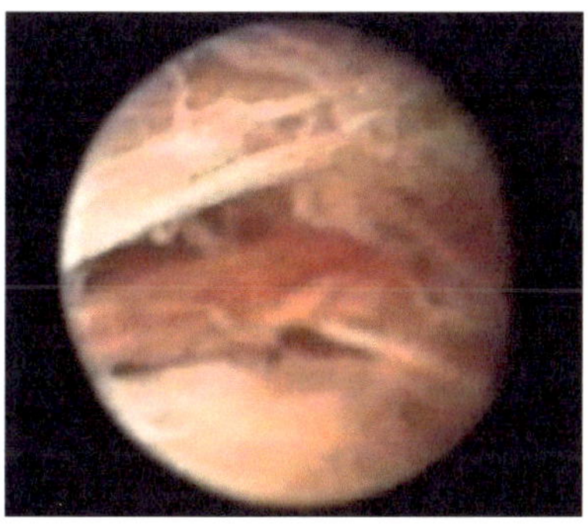

Figure 20. Posterior recess of the superior compartment of the left TMJ. Eburneation of glenoid fossa, adhesions and fibrillations with „crab meat" appearance, mild granulations, irregularities of condylar surface, hyperaemia of the posterior attachment can be determined. Some debris is visible in the superior aspect of the field.

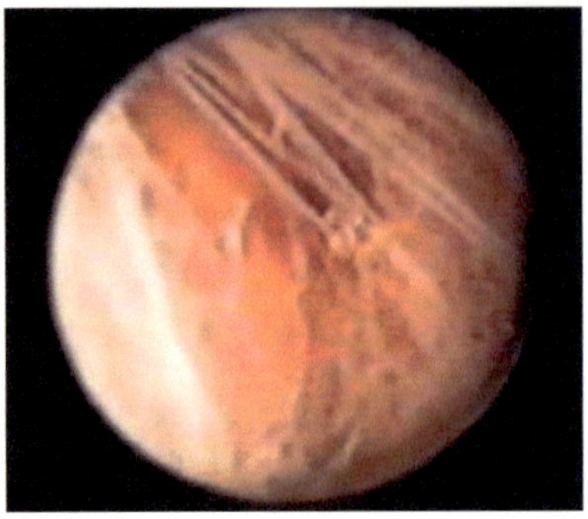

Figure 21. Posterior recess of the superior compartment of the right TMJ. The irregular surface of the remodeled retrodiscal tissues, fibrous adhesions, fibrillations and smooth fibres seen clearly. Synovial inflammation is obvious, localizing in the posterior part of the disc. Some loose bodies (chondromatosis granules) are detectable.

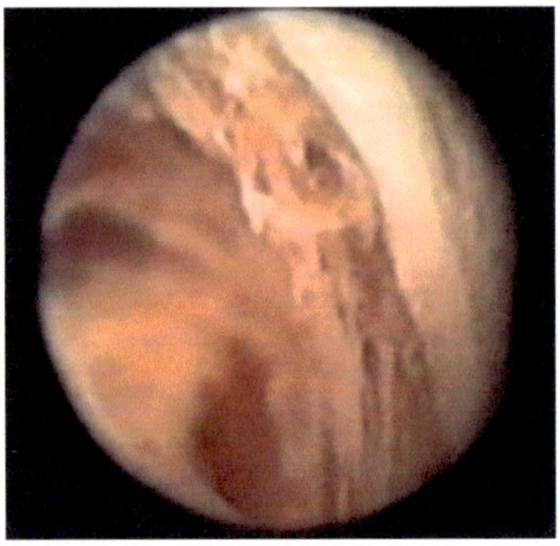

(a)

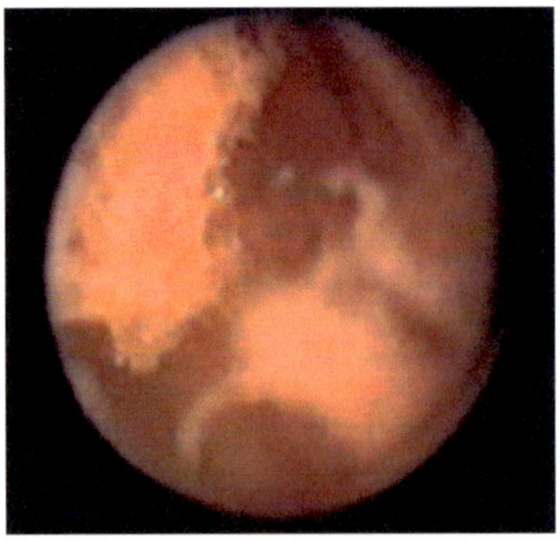

(b)

Figure 22. a. Posterior recess of the superior compartment of the left TMJ. Debris on the posterior glenoid fossa wall can be seen. Fibrillations, adhesions and increased vascularization in the posterior capsular wall. b. Posterior recess of the superior compartment of the left TMJ. Hyperaemia in the posterior capsular wall. A greater amount of floating debris and some granules (foreign bodies) are noted.

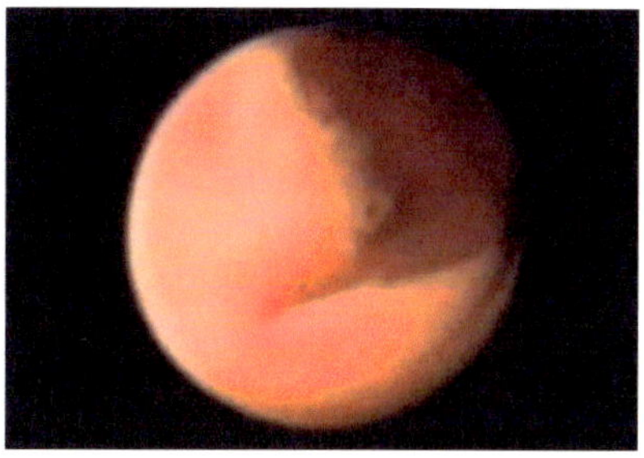

Figure 23. Appearance of the superior compartment of the TMJ after arthroscopic debridement. The apparent intimate relationship of the glenoid fossa with the valley of the retrodiscal tissue and its junction with the disc in an essentially normal TMJ. The joint space is free of debris.

The patients are to be followed up after 6 months and approximayely 5 years after the operation. Intravenous antibiotics at the beginning of the procedure is recommended. Concepts of irrigation are to maintain the capsule distended through the procedure. Continuous irrigation constantly cleanses a joint debris and blood, increases mobility, reliefing symptoms. It is also important to use of adjunctive therapy postoperatively to obtain maximum success with arthroscopic surgery *e.g.* physical therapy especially in case of haemorrage, as it may prolong healing time *e.g.* ultrasound with hydrocortisone ointment. A pressure dressing during the first couple of hours after the operation is recommended.

6.5. Summary of arthroscopic findings

Arthroscopic findings included surface adhesions, stickness of the superior surface of the disc to the anterior fossa portion and articular eminence, superior compartment adhesions, anteromedially displaced disc without reduction and morphologic changes in the disc. A number of arthroscopic findings as fibrous adherences mainly between the disc and fossa, fibrillations with „crab meat" appearance, mild granulations, irregularities of condylar surface, foreign bodies, increased vascularisation are to be found. Synovitis in the upper joint space of the TMJ has been observed during arthroscopy and this inflamed synovium may cause pain. The alterations in the constituents of the synovial fluid affect lubrication of the joint causing stickness and decreased mobility. Synovial chondromatosis has been found in the joint space [10, 45,46]. Synovial chondromatosis of the TMJ in both the superior and inferior joint compartments have found due to osteoarthritis during long period ~ 10 years [47].

6.6. Complications

Intra- and postoperative complications for arthroscopy are rare. Bleeding may be from branches of the temporal vein during puncture. Extravasation of irrigation fluid into surrounding tissues may be occur sometimes due to leakage of the irrigating fluid into the surrounding tissues caused by accidental perforation of the TMJ capsule. This situation is easily controled if the surgeon always check the out-flow from out-flow cannula. From postoperative complications a few cases with otologic complications and nerve damage have been reported

[5,48]. Injurie of superficial branches of facial nerve resulting to paraesthesia in the preauricular region was observed in two cases. These symptoms disappeared during one month [10].

7. Analysis of clinical data and results

It has been shown that during arthroscopy several inflammatory and pain mediators causing destructive changes, foreign bodies as grains of chondromatosis are washed out elicitating joint noises [9,49]. For the patients with episodic signs and symptoms a noninvasive conservative approach is indicated (Wilkies stages I-III). Procedures currently used for the TMJ derangements as osteoarthritis/arthrosis (Wilkies stages IV and V) are: arthrocentesis, arthroscopy, arthrotomy or TMJ replacement. From arthroscopic findings fibrillation seemed to be the most common ~76% [50]. Arthroscopic lysis and lavage has been an effective treatment for TMJ disorders refractory to nonsurgical treatments [8,12,51]. An evaluation following temporomandibular joint arthroscopic surgery with lysis and lavage after 2 to 10,8 years treatment showed that arthroscopic surgery of the temporomandibular joint is successful in the long term for patients with painful motion [11,52]. Assessment of symptoms reported by the patient as well as of objective signs noted on clinical examination confirms resolution of pain on movement and increased vertical opening.

A significant and maintained improvement in MIO and VAS is also observed over the 5 years period of time (Figure 24, 25) [10].

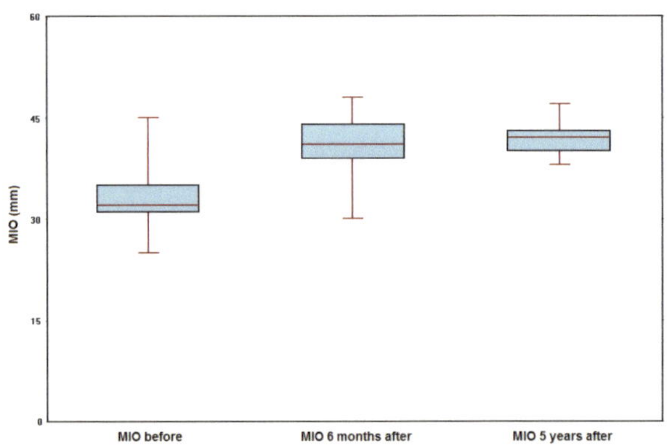

Figure 24. Graphical representation of VAS values (median) before treatment and after 6 months and 5 years treatment in patients (n = 29).

TMJ arthroscopy is especially useful when the disc has not yet been deformed. Superior joint compartment adhesions and disc immobility can be treated during arthroscopic procedure, leading to resolution of symptoms and return of joint function [10]. The adhesions may cause retention of the disc in its anteriorly displaced position, which may explain the failure to

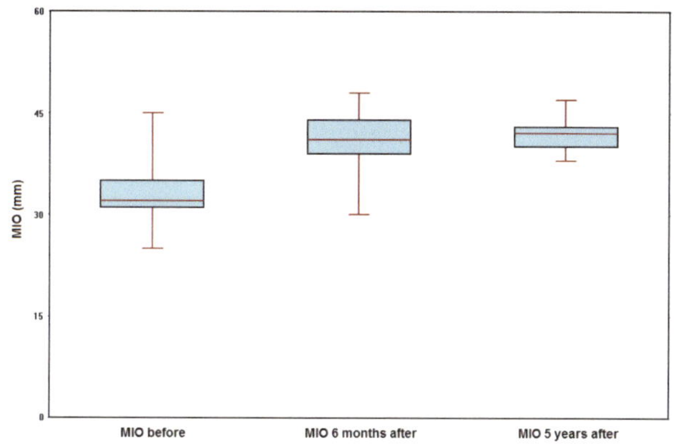

Figure 25. Graphical representation of MIO values (median) before treatment and after 6 months and 5 years after treatment in patients (n = 29).

respond to conservative treatment. An adherence of the disc to the fossa may be caused by an alteration of the normal lubrication of the joint as a result of intermittent joint overloading, with secondary activation of oxidative species and degradation of hyaluronic acid. Anchored Disc Phenomen could be one of the first clinical symptoms observed in the chain events that would end in a more severe internal derangement [52, 53].

Long-term results of TMJ arthroscopy have been analysed demonstrating a high accuracy for adhesions, fibrillations and degenerative changes of the bone structures. The adhesions may cause retention of the disc in its anteriorly displaced position, which may explain the failing response to conservative treatment. It has been shown that during this procedure several inflammatory and pain mediators causing destructive changes and granules of chondromatosis are washed out elicitating joint noises [10, 22, 40]. It is important to select the procedure with the highest probability of success and least morbidity. For the patients with episodic signs and symptoms a noninvasive, conservative approach is indicated (Wilkies stages I-III). Procedures currently used for the TMJ derangements as osteoarthritis/arthrosis (Wilkies stages IV and V) are: arthrocentesis [12], arthroscopy, arthrotomy or TMJ replacement [5,54]. Pain and hypomobility seems to be a part of a wide spectrum of symptoms appearing in the context of chronic dysfunction of the TMJ. Some authors have reported that the major symptom has been closed lock phenomenon [12,55]. From arthroscopic findings [55] fibrillation seemed to be the most common -76%. In other study [10] closed lock was found in 17,2 % and fibrillations in 75,8 % of cases. Arthroscopic lysis and lavage has been an effective treatment for TMJ disorders refractory to nonsurgical treatments [8,12,51]. Several authors [52] performed long-term evaluation following temporomandibular joint arthroscopic surgery with lysis and lavage after 2 to 10,8 years treatment. On the bases of assessment of symptoms reported by the patients as well as objective signs noted on clinical examination confirmed resolution of pain on movement and increased vertical opening. In a later study also lysis and lavage improved translation of the joint, decreased or eliminated pain.

The chief presenting complaint for most patients (86,2%) was pain preoperatively. A significant maintained decrease in VAS score was achieved after 6 months and also 5 years follow-up. A significant and maintained improvement in MIO was also observed over the same period of time [10]. The results are comparable to those reported in the other papers [34,52]. It is important to take into account that the sympathetic and sensory nerve fibres within the temporomandibular joint are located in the anterior recess and the retrodiscal tissue of the upper compartment. Anterior disc release may reduce the number of these nerve fibres in arthroscopic procedures, thus influencing pain dynamics. The advantages of arthroscopy compared with open joint surgery using the Jaw Pain and Function Questionnaire are that arthroscopic surgery is less invasive and associated with lower morbidity [15]. No statistical differences were also observed between arthroscopic lysis and lavage and operative arthroscopy in relation to postoperative pain or MIO at any stage of the follow-up period [9]. Arthroscopic lysis and lavage has been found effective in 84% of patients in case of osteoarthritis of TMJ [55]. Multiple adhesions also develop skeletal changes, with a shortened ramus. If the condition develops rapidly enough, open bite and rethrognathia may occur [40,56,57]. During arthroscopic surgery nodules of TMJ synovial chondromatosis are able to pass through the cannula by lavage with saline solution [49].

An adherence of the disc to the fossa may be caused by an alteration of the normal lubrication of the joint as a result of intermittent joint overloading, with secondary activation of oxidative species and degradation of hyaluronic acid. Anchored Disc Phenomen could be one of the first clinical symptoms observed in the chain events that would end in a more severe internal derangement [52,53].

Based on the present findings, it follows that a displaced disc, by itself, is of only limited significance.This is not surprising because the majority of individuals with derangement of the TMJ are asymptomatic [7,57]. The intriguing question that remains is why lavage and lysis of adhesions or high-pressure irrigation of the upper joint space should be therapeutic. The answer is, that during this procedure several inflammatory mediators available in the synovial fluid as prostaglandins [58], cytokines [22,59], serotonin as pain mediator [28] etc. are washed out. In episodes of closed lock, the limitation in condylar movement probably originates from changes in the upper compartment that restrict the sliding motion of the disc; This course of events may explain the efficacy of lysis and lavage of only this joint space, as this manipulation allows translation of the disc along the eminence, allowing the condyle to complete its natural path. The data in the literature have stated that the most frequent disc displacements were anterior and anteromedial [52].

In episodes of closed lock, the limitation in condylar movement probably originates from the changes in the upper compartment that restrict the sliding motion of the disc. The data in the literature have stated that the most frequent disc displacements were anterior and anteromedial [39,60]. Using MRI pre- and postoperatively revealed that disc position remained anteriorly without reduction, disc mobility increased after arthroscopic surgery[8]. Improvement in joint symptoms and function is not attributed so much as to the restoration of disc position as to possible release of the lateral capsular fibrosis during arthroscopy [52,61].

http://dx.doi.org/10.5772/55011

8. Arthrotomy

Arthrotomy can play an important role in the management of the TMJ disorders. There are conditions that require primary surgical management as developmental disturbances (condylar hypo-, hyperplasia of the mandible, tumours, ankylosis etc.). Secondary surgical management is indicated in case of arthritis, disc displacements, trauma, synovial chondromatosis. Not treated properly and immediately a juvenile trauma to the TMJ area can lead to ankylosis. Arthrotomy has been recognised as the only treatment method of fibrous or osseous ankylosis.There is still a group of patients whom an arthrotomy and disc surgery are necessary *e.g.* to treat painful clicking in patients with anteriorly displaced, nonreducing discs and limited mouth opening, irreparable disc perforation or if it is misshaped, shortened, rigid. Large medial osteophyts on the condyle are very difficult to shave arthroscopically, and in these situations they are better to handle *via* arthrotomy (Figure 26).

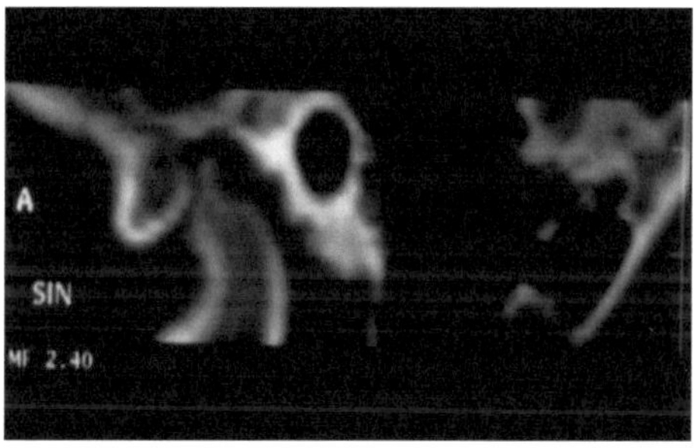

Figure 26. An osteophyte in the medial part of the right mandibular condyle in a sagittal view of the CT. Cortical destruction of the glenoid fossa surface.

Large central cartilaginous perforations may need an arthrotomy and possibly discectomy, although there are data about healing of disk perforations as the bilaminar zone undergoes metaplastic changes forming pseudodisc [61]. The importance of disc position and shape is emphasized by many authors [8, 51]. As a result, open joint procedures are developed to reposition the displaced disc [7, 9]. A surgical procedure for TMJ disc-repositioning surgery using bioresorbable fixation screws for stabilisation of the disc to the condyle is reported [62], but the efficacy of the method described should be confirmed by the long-term studies. Arthrotomy includes not only a discoplasty but also high condylar shave and eminectomy. For discectomy the medial disc attachment is cut with curved scissors, facilitating approach to the lower joint space. Direct comparison of the clinical results are achieved in patients following arthroscopic surgery with a group of patients who underwent open surgery. The postoperative follow-up period ranged 5 to 6 years and 9 months. These results following open and arthroscopic surgery measured with the Jaw Pain and Function Questionnaire a self rating scale, originally published by Clark et al. [17] and differentiated by Wilkes′ stages. No significant difference was noted when comparing the group 5 years postoperatively [15]. Some patients with a presentation of TMJ pathology however, have a history of previous mandibular trauma. Following trauma a joint ankylosis may occur. Ankylosis is more likely in younger patients and it can be also classified as true and false. False ankylosis results from pathologic conditions not directly related to the joint (Figure 27).

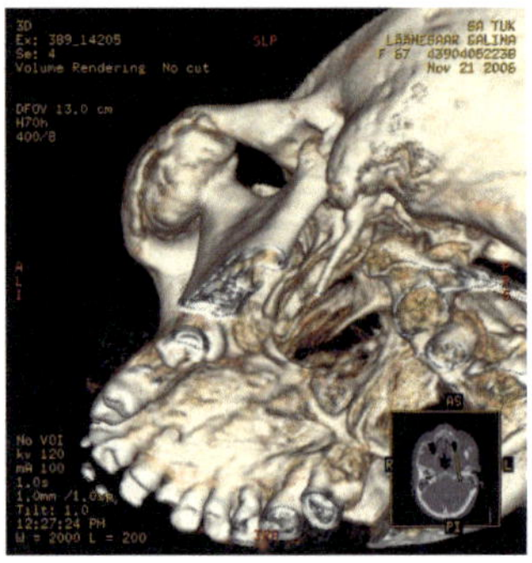

Figure 27. CT 3D reconstruction of the false ankylosis resulting from the osteochondroma of the left coronoid process.

There are several things to be considered the traumatically induced ankylosis. TMJ is commonly traumatized indirectly by blows to the mandible. It is known, that at least 35% of mandibular fractures involve the condyle [63]. It is found, that in 64% of the ankylosis cases, the patients had fractures of the mandible locating in the anterior area of the mandible and they were not diagnosed in time or not treated properly [65]. Synovial chondromatosis (SC) of the TMJ is a rare benign condition characterized by the formation of metaplastic cartilage in the synovium resulting in osteocartilagenous loose bodies within the joint [65]. We have analysed arthroscopic findings and synovial chondromatosis was observed in 17% of cases of treated patients due to TMJ osteoarthritis [10]. Differential diagnosis is necessary to perform with calcium pyrophosphate dihydrate crystal deposition disease of the TMJ.

8.1. Method of arthrotomy

Under general anaesthesia and naso-tracheal intubation (with fibre endoscope if necessary), a preauricular incision is performed. Preauricular approach is the most commonly used to expose the TMJ. Once the incision is carried through the skin and subcutaneous tissues, the tissue layer, containing partly the parotid gland, facial nerve branches, auriculotemporal nerve, superficial temporal artery and vein is bluntly reflected forward with the elevator in order to expose the joint capsule. Then a vertical incision is made to begin to expose the joint space (Figure 28, 29). After performing arthroplasty the wound can be closed in the usual fashion.

http://dx.doi.org/10.5772/55011

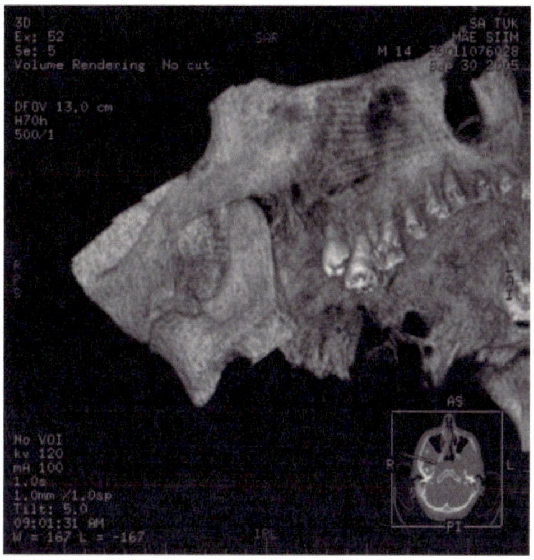

Figure 28. D image of the CT showing fibroosseous ankylosis of the right TMJ on a 15 yrs. boy. Trauma took place at the age of 4 years.

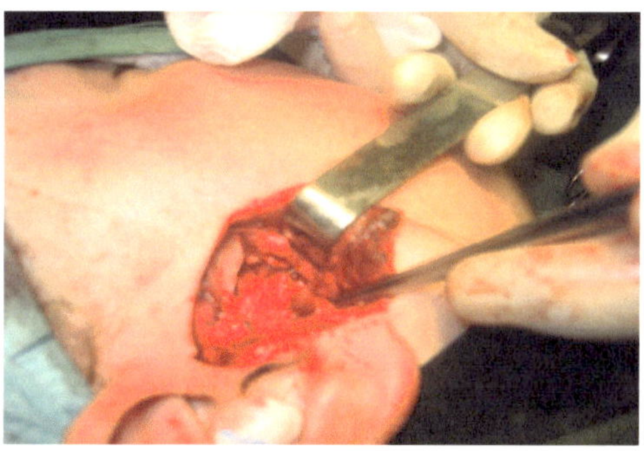

Figure 29. Arthrotomy of the same 15 yrs boy is performed. The right ankylotic TMJ is exposed.

We have used [66] the suture anchor in interpositional arthroplasty in case of the temporomandibular joint ankylosis traumatic origin. Ankylotic left TMJ was exposed and a gap arthroplasty was performed using different types of burs. An ipsilateral myofascial temporal pedicled flap was prepared, rotated inferiorly and interposed between the head of the condyle and the mandibular fossa.. The mini anchor in the lateral pole of the condyle was inserted and anchored suture of the myofascial flap was performed and the capsule was sutured.(Figure 30a, 30b, 31a, 31b, 32).

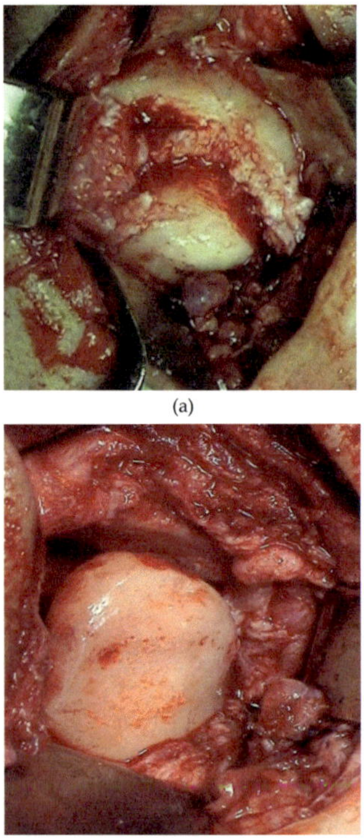

(a)

(b)

Figure 30. a. Ankylotic left TMJ is exposed for osteotomy. b. The osseous components of the TMJ after arthroplasty and the joint space is formed.

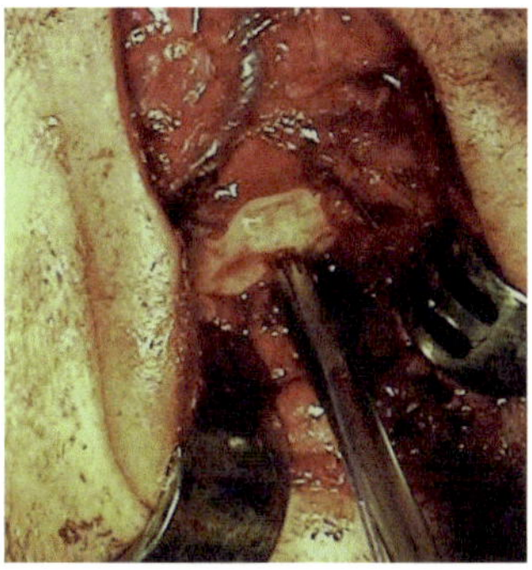

(a)

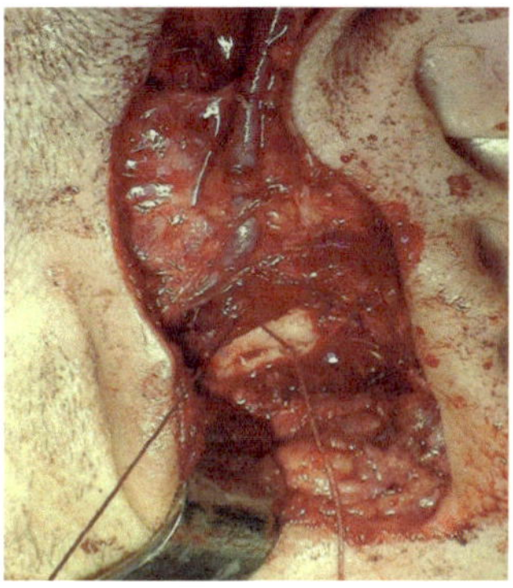

(b)

Figure 31. a. Insertion of the mini anchore in the lateral pole of the condyle. b. The condyle and the anchored suturing of the myofascial flap.

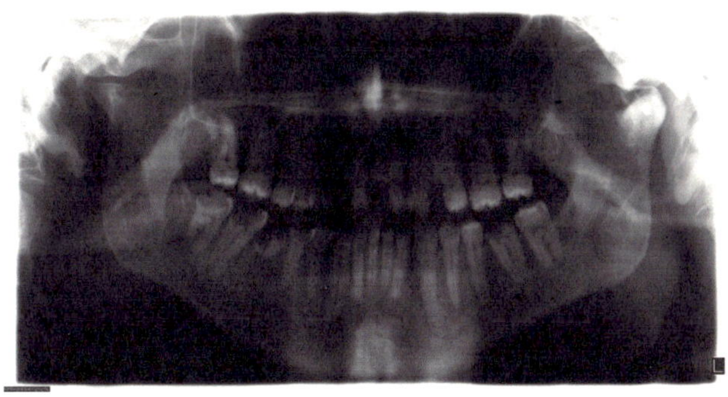

Figure 32. Post-operative ortopantomograph showing an acceptable anatomy of the left mandibular condyle and articular fossa and a formed space between them.The mini anchor is visualized in the condyle.

The standard treatment in case of synovial chondromatosis is arthrotomy of the affected joint and removal of the loose bodies. In our case granular masses with different size situated in the upper compartment of the TMJ (Figure33, 34, 35a). Histological findings showed chondrometaplasia of the synovial membrane (Figure 35b) [67]. Arthroscopy is proved to be useful for management of synovial chondromatosis of the TMJ in case of granules smaller than 3 mm which are commonly removed with joint lavage [10]. OPTG and CT scans reveale usually calcifying lesions in the TMJ region.

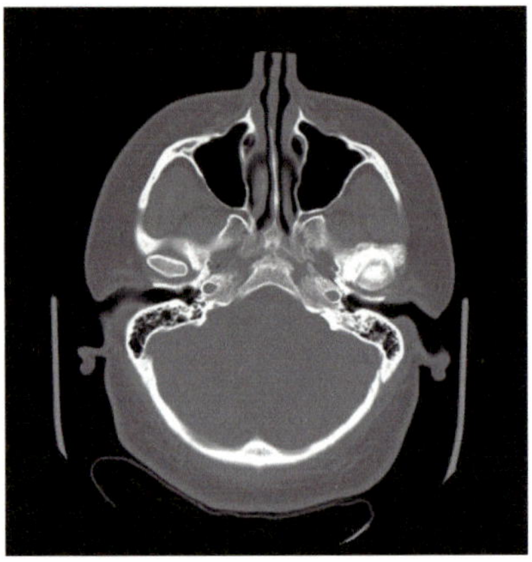

Figure 33. Axial view of the CT scan of the patient (female, 44 yrs.), showing granular masses surrounding the left condylar head.

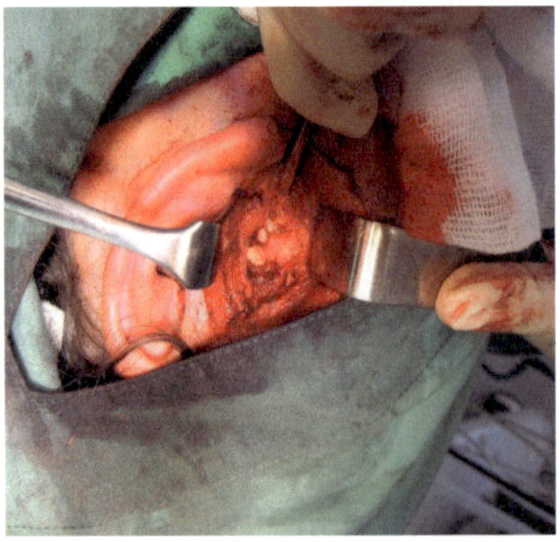

Figure 34. Intra-operative finding of the same patient (female, 44 yrs.) with irregular cartilaginous loose granules in the posterior recess of the upper compartment of the TMJ.

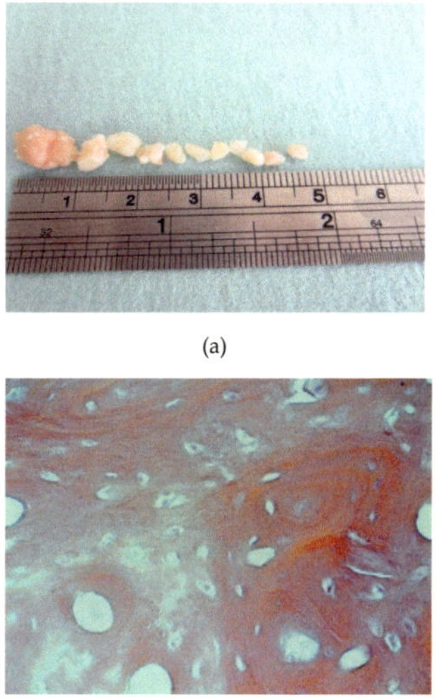

(a)

(b)

Figure 35. a. The different size of granules are pearly white, of varying shape and ranging in the size from 3,0 to 10,0 mm.b. Histologically clustered hyaline chondrocytes with synovial lining are visible. Staining with haematoxylin-eosin, magnification 40X.

9. Summary

Early diagnosis is the key to successful treatment, because it permits the use of nonsurgical means or minimally invasive procedures (arthrocentesis, arthroscopy). In late stage disease is indicated arthrotomy, to attain an improved quality of life with less pain and improved function. Clinical success of arthroscopy is based on several factors. Lysis and lavage remove intraarticular inflammatory and pain mediators. The release of fibrillations and adhearences as well as improvement in discal mobility allows to distrbute the functional stresses on the articular tissues and adverse loading on the joints is decreased. The long-term outcome of TMJ arthroscopic surgery with lysis and lavage is considered to be acceptable and effective. Fibrillations and fibrous adhesions are the most usual pathological signs of arthroscopic findings in patients with internal derangement of the TMJ. Arthroscopic releasing of these restrictive bands improves the joint mobility and contributes to reducing pain level. The results of arthroscopy offered favourable long-term stable results with regard to increasing MIO and reducing pain and dysfunction. The improvement in joint mobility and disc mobility will lead to adaptive changes in the hard tissues.This may implay that the arthroscopic procedure with mechanics may stop the process of further TMJ degeneration. The advantages of arthroscopy compared with open joint surgery are that arthroscopic surgery is less invasive, procedure needs less time and associated with lower morbidity. Arthrotomy is indicated in cases with anteriorly displaced, nonreducing discs who continue to have pain and limited mouth opening despite the treatment by either arthrocentesis or arthroscopic surgery that has not responded to arthrocentesis or arthroscopy. In conclusion procedures such as arthrocentesis, arthroscopic surgery and arthrotomy can be used with reasonably good results in properly selected cases.

Acknowledgements

The publication of this chapter is supported by Ernst Jaakson Memorial Scholarship.

Author details

Edvitar Leibur[1,2], Oksana Jagur[1] and Ülle Voog-Oras[1]

1 Department of Stomatology, Tartu University, Tartu University Hospital, Estonia

2 Department of Internal Medicine, Tartu University, Tartu University Hospital, Estonia

References

[1] Sanders B, Buonocristiani R.Diagnostic and Surgical Arthroscopy of the Temporomandibular Joint: Clinical Experience with 137 Procedures over a 2-year period. Journal of Craniomandibular Disorders: Facial & Oral Pain 1987;12(3) 202-213.

[2] Tag H. Arthroscope. Journal of Japanese Orthopedic Association 1939;14, 359-362.

[3] Onishi M. Arthroscopy of the temporomandibular joint (author´s transl.). Journal of Japanese Stomatological Association 1975;(42) 207-213.

[4] Onishi M. Clinical application arthroscopy in the temporomandibular joint diseases. Bulletin Tokyo Medical Dental University 1980;(27) 141-148.

[5] McCain JP, Sanders B, Koslin MG, Quinn JH, Peters PB, Indresano AT. Temporomandibular joint arthroscopy : a 6-year multicenter retrospective study of 4,831 joints. Journal of Oral and Maxillofacial Surgery 2002;50(9) 926-930.

[6] Holmlund AB, Axelsson S.Temporomandibular arthropathy: correlation between clinical signs and symptoms and arthroscopic findings. International Journal of Oral & Maxillofacial Surgery 1996;25(3) 266-271.

[7] Holmlund AB, Axelsson S,Gynther GW. A comparison of discectomy and arthroscopic lysis and lavage for the treatment of chronic closed lock of the temporomandibular joint: a randomized outcome study. Journal of Oral and Maxillofacial Surgery 2001;59(9) 972-977.

[8] Ohnuki T, Fukuda M, Iino M, Takahahshi T. Magnetic resonance evaluation of the disk before and after arthroscopic surgery for temporomandibular disorders. Oral

Surgery Oral Medicine Oral Pathology Oral Radiology Endodontics 2003;96(2) 141-148.

[9] González-Garcia R, Rodriguez-Campo FJ, Monje F, Sastre-Perez J, Gil-Diez Usandizaga JL. Operative versus simple arthroscopic surgery for chronic closed lock of the temporomandibular joint: a clinical study of 344 arthroscopic procedures. International Journal of Oral&Maxillofacial Surery 2008;17(9) 790-796.

[10] Leibur E, Jagur O, Müürsepp P, Veede L, Voog-Oras Ü. Long-term evaluation of arthroscopic surgery with lysis and lavage of temporomandibular disorders. Journal of Cranio-Maxillo-Facial Surgery 2010;38(8) 615-620.

[11] Murakami K, Segami N, Okamoto I, Takahashi K,Tsuboi, Y. Outcome of arthroscopic surgery for internal derangement of the temporomandibular joint: long – term results covering 10 years. Journal of Cranio-Maxillo-Facial Surgery 2000;28(3) 264 – 271.

[12] Sanroman JF. Closed lock (MRI fixed disc): a comparison of arthrocentesis and arthroscopy. International Journal of Oral & Maxillofacial Surgery 2004;33(4) 344-348.

[13] Mancha de la Plata M, Muñoz-Guerra M, Escorial Hernandez V, Martos Diaz P, Gil-Diez Usandizaga JL, Rodriguez-Campo FJ. Unsuccessful temporomandibular joint arthroscopy: is a second arthroscopy an acceptable alternative? Journal of Oral and Maxillofacial Surgery 2008;66(10) 2086-2092.

[14] Voog Ü, Alstergren P, Leibur E, Kallikorm R, Kopp S. Impact of temporomandibular joint pain on activities of daily living in patients with rheumatoid arthritis. Acta Odontologica Scandinavica 2003;61(5) 278-282.

[15] Undt G, Murakami KI, Rasse M, Ewers R. Open versus arthroscopic surgery for internal derangement of the temporomandibular joint: A retrospective study comparing two centers results using Jaw Pain and Function Questionnaire. Journal of Cranio-Maxillo-Facial Surgery 2006;34(4) 234-241.

[16] Jagur O, Kull M, Leibur E, Kallikorm R, Loorits D, Lember M,Voog-Oras Ü. The associations of TMJ pain and bone characteristics on the activities of daily living. Open Journal of Stomatology 2012 (accepted for publication).

[17] Clark GT, Seligman D, Solberg WK, Pullinger AG. Guidlines for the examination and diagnosis of temporomandibular disorders. Journal of Craniomandibular Disorders 1989;3(1) 7-14.

[18] Sommer OJ, Aigner F, Rudisch A, Gruber H, Fritsch H, Millesi W, Stiskal M. Cross-sectional and Functional Images of the Temporomandibular Joint: Radiology, Pathology, and Basic Biomechanics of the Jaw Radiographics. Radiology 2003;23(6) 428-432.

[19] Schmelzle R. Lokalanästhesie. In: Zahnärztliche Chirurgie. 2. Auflage Urban & Schwarzenberg. München-Wien-Baltimore1989; p.19.

[20] Tallents RH, MacherDJ, Kyrkanides S, Katzberg RW, Moss M.E. Prevalence of mising posterior teeth and intraarticular temporomandibular disorders. Journal of Prosthetic Dentistry 2002;87(1) 45-49.

[21] Voog Ü, Alstergren P, Eliasson S, Leibur E, Kallikorm R, Kopp S.Progression of radiographic changes in the temporomandibular joints of patients with rheumatoid arthritis in relation to inflammatory markers and mediators in the blood. Acta Odontologica Scandinavica 2004;62(1) 7-13.

[22] Voog Ü, Alstergren P, Eliasson S, Leibur E, Kallikorm R, Kopp S. Inflammatory mediators and radiographic changes in temporomandibular joints in patients with rheumatoid arthritis. Acta Odontologica Scandinavica 2003;61(1) 57-64.

[23] Kim SJ, Park YH, Hong SP, Cho BO, Park JW, Kim SG. The presence of bacteria in the synovial fluid of the temporomandibular joint and clinical significance: preliminary study. Journal of Oral and Maxillofacial Surgery 2003;61(10) 1156-1161.

[24] Paegle DI, Holmlund AB, öStlund MR, Grillner L. The occurence of Antibodies against Chlamydia species in patients with monoarthritis and chronic closed lock of the temporomandibular joint. Journal of Oral and Maxillofacial Surgery 2004;62(4) 435-439.

[25] Alstergren P, Kopp S, Theodorson E. Synovial fluid sampling from the temporomandibular joint: sample quality criteria and levels of interleukin-1 beta and serotonin. Acta Odontologica Scandinavica 1999;57(1) 278-282.

[26] Kamada A, Kakudo K, Arika T, Okazaki J, Kano M, Sakaki T. Assay of synovial MMP3 in temporomandibular joint diseases. Journal of Cranio-Maxillo- Facial Surgery 2000;28(3) 247-248.

[27] Alstergren P, Kopp S. Pain and synovial fluid concentration in arthritic temporomandibular joints. Pain 2007;2(1-2) 137-143.

[28] Voog Ü, Alstergren P, Leibur E, Kallikorm R, Kopp S. Immediate effect of the serotonin antagonist granisetron on temporomandibular joint pain in patients with systemic inflammatory disorders. Life Sciences 2000;68(5) 591-602.

[29] Warden SJ, Haney EM. Skeletal effects of serotonin (5-hydroxytryptamine) transporter inhibition: evidence from in vitro and animal-based studies. Journal of Musculoskeletal Neuronal Interaction 2008;8(2) 121-132.

[30] Wilkes CH. Internal derangements of the temporomandibular joint. Pathological variations. Archives of Otolaryngology, Head Neck Surgery 1989;115(4) 469-477.

[31] List T, Helkimo M. A scale for measuring the activities of daily living (ADL) of patients with craniomandibular disorders. Swedish Dental Journal 1995;19(1) 33-40.

[32] Kaselo E, Jagomägi T,Voog U. Malocclusion and the need for orthodontic treatment in patients with temporomandibular dysfunction. Stomatologija. Baltic Dental and Maxillofacial Journal 2007;9(3) 79-85.

[33] Whyte AM, McNamara D, Rosenberg I,Whyte AW. Magnetic resonance imaging in the evaluation of temporomandibular joint disc displacement. International Journal of Oral & Maxillofacial Surgery 2006;35(8) 696-703.

[34] Landes CA, Goral WA, Sader R, Mack MG. 3-D sonography for diagnosis of disc dislocation of the temporomandibular joint compared with MRI. Ultrasound Medical Biology 2007;32(5) 633-639.

[35] Rohlin M, Ăkerman S,Kopp S. Tomography as an aid to detect macroscopic changes of the temporomandibular joint . Acta Odontologica Scandinavica 1986;44(3) 131-140.

[36] Helenius L, Hallikainen D, Meurman J, Koskimies S, Tervahartiala P, Kivisaari L, Hietanen J, Suuronen R, Lindqvist C, Leirisalo-Repo M. HLA-DRB1* alleles and temporomandibular joint erosion in patients with rheumatic disease. Scandinavian Journal of Rheumatology 2004;33(1) 24-29.

[37] Suarez FR, Bhussry BR, Neff PA, Huang HK,Vaughn D. A preliminary study of computerized tomographs of the temporomandibular joint. The Compendium on continuing education in general dentistry 1980;1(3) 217-222.

[38] Raustia M, Pyhtinen J, Virtanen KK. Examination of the temporomandibular joint by direct sagittal computed tomography. Clinical Radiology 1985;36(3) 291-296.

[39] Larheim TA,Westesson P, Sano T. Temporomandibular Joint Disk Displacement: Comparison in Asymptomatic Volunteers and Patients. Radiology 2001;218(2) 428-32.

[40] Emshoff R, Brandlmaier I, Bertram S, Rudish A.Relative odds of temporomandibular joint pain as a function of magnetic resonance imaging findings of internal derangement, osteoarthrosis, effusion, and bone marrow edema. Oral Surgery Oral Medicine Oral Pathology Oral Radiology Endodontics 2003;95(4) 437-445.

[41] Rohlin M, Petersson A. Rheumatoid arthritis of the temporomandibular joint: radiologic evaluation based on standard reference films. Oral Surgery, Oral Medicine, and Oral Pathology 1989;67(5) 594-599.

[42] Gaggle A, Schults G, Santler G, Kärcher H, Simbrunner J. Clinical and magnetic resonance findings in the temporomandibular joints of patients before and after ortognathic surgery. The British Journal of Oral & Maxillofacial Surgery 1999;37(1) 41-45.

[43] Landes C, Walendzik H, Klein C. Sonography of the temporomandibular joint from 60 examinations and comparison with MRI and axiography. Journal of Cranio-Maxillo-Facial Surgery 2000;28(6) 352-361.

[44] Torres DE, McCain JP. Arthroscopic elrctrothermal capsulorrhaphy for the treatment of recurrent temporomandibular joint dislocation. International Journal of Oral & Maxillofacial Surgery 2012;41(6) 681-689.

[45] Mercuri LG. Synovial chondromatosis of the temporomandibular joint with medial cranial fossa extension. International Journal of Oral & Maxillofacial Surgery 2008;37(7) 684-685.

[46] González-Pérez LM, Concregado-Córdoba J, Salinas-Martin MV. Temporomandibular joint synovial chondromatosis with a traumatic etiology. International Journal of Oral & Maxillofacial Surgery 2011;40(3) 330-334.

[47] Sato J, Segami N, Suzuki T, Yoshitake Y, Nishikawa K.The expression of fibroblast growth factor receptor 1 in chondrocytes in synovial chondromatosis of the temporomandibular joint. Report of two cases. International Journal of Oral & Maxillofacial Surgery 2002;31(7) 532-536.

[48] Appelbaum EL, Berg LF, Kumar A, Mafee MF. Otologic complications Following temporomandibular joint arthroscopy. Annals of Otology, Rhinology, Laryngology 1988;97(6) 675-679.

[49] Shibuya T, Kino K, Yoshida S, Amagasa T.Arthroscopic removal of nodules of synovial chondromatosis of the temporomandibular joint. Cranio 2002;20(4) 304-306.

[50] Dimitroulis G. A review of 56 cases of chronic closed lock treated with temporomandibular joint arthroscopy. Journal of Oral and Maxillofacial Surgery 2002;60(5) 519-524.

[51] Politi M, Sembronio S, Robiony M, Costa F, Toro C, Undt G. High condylectomy and disc repositioning compared to arthroscopic lysis, lavage and capsular strech for the treatment of chronic closed lock of the temporomandibular joint. Oral Surgery Oral Medicine Oral Pathology Oral Radiology Endodontics 2007;103(1) 27 - 33.

[52] Sorel B, Piecuch JF. Long-term evaluation following temporomandibular joint arthroscopy with lysis and lavage. International Journal of Oral & Maxillofacial Surgery 2000;29(4) 532-536.

[53] Krug J, Jirousek Z, Suchmova H, Germakova E. Influence of discoplasty and discectomy of the temporomandibular joint on elimination of pain and restricted mouth opening. Acta Medica (Hradec Kralove) 2004;47(1) 47-53.

[54] Smolka W, Iizuka T. Arthroscopic lysis and lavage in different stages of internal derangement of the temporomandibular joint: correlation of preoperative staging to arthroscopic findings and treatment outcome. Journal of Oral and Maxillofacial Surgery 2005;63(4) 471-478.

[55] Dimitroulis G. The prevalence of osteoarthrosis in cases of advanced internal derangement of the Temporomandibular Joint: a clinical, surgical and histological study. International Journal of Oral & Maxillofacial Surgery 2005;34(2) 345-349.

[56] Emshoff R. Clinical factors affecting the outcome of arthrocentesis and hydraulic distension of the temporomandibular joint. Oral Surgery Oral Medicine Oral Pathology Oral Radiology Endodontics 2005;100(4) 409-414.

[57] Hamada Y, Kondoh T, Holmlund AB, Iino M, Kobayashi K, Seto K.Influence of arthroscopically observed fibrous adhesions before and after joint irrigation on clinical outcome in patients with chronic closed lock of the temporomandibular joint. International Journal of Oral & Maxillofacial Surgery 2005; 34(7) 727-732.

[58] Murakami KI, Shibata T, Kubota E, Maeda H. Intra-articular levels of prostaglandin E_2 , hyaluronic acid, and chondroitin -4 and -6 sulfates in the temporomandibular joint synovial fluid of patients with internal derangement. Journal of Oral and Maxillofacial Surgery 1998;56(2) 199-203.

[59] Kardel R, Ulfgren AK, Reinholt FP, Holmlund A. Inflammatory cell and cytokine patterns in patients with painful clicking and osteoarthritis in the temporomandibular joint. International Journal of Oral & Maxillofacial Surgery 2003;32(5) 390-396.

[60] Güven O. Management of chronic recurrent temporomandibular joint dislocations: A retrospective study. Journal of Craniomaxillofacial Surgery 2009;37(1) 24-29.

[61] Moses JJ, Lo H. The treatment of internal derangement of the temporomandibular joint – an arthroscopic approach. Oral Surgery Oral Diagnosis 1992;.3, 5-11.

[62] Sembronio S, Robiony M, Politi M. Disc-repositioning surgery of the temporomandibular joint using bioresorbable screws. International Journal of Oral & Maxillofacial Surgery 2006;35(10) 1149-1152.

[63] Bradley P. Injuries of the condylar region and coronal process. In Rowe NL, Williams JL (eds.): Maxillofacial Injuries, Vol.1. London, England, Churchill Livingstone, 1985, pp. 337-339

[64] He D, Ellis E. 3rd., Zhang Y. Etiology of temporomandibular joint ankylosis secondary to condylar fractures: the role of concomitant mandibular fractures. Journal of Oral and Maxillofacial Surgery 2008;66(1).74-78

[65] Ardekian L, Faquin W, Troulis M, Kaban LB, August M. Synovial chondromatosis of the temporomandibular joint: report and analysisof eleven cases. Journal of Oral and Maxillofacial Surgery 2005;63,(5) 941-947.

[66] Nestal-Zibo H, Leibur E, Voog Oras Ü, Tamme T. Use of the suture anchor in interpositional arthroplasty of temporomandibular joint ankylosis. Oral and Maxillofacial Surgery 2012;16(1) 157-162.

[67] Jagur O, Leibur E, Erm T. Synovial chondromatosis of the temporomandibular joint. A case report. Stomatologija. Baltic Dental and Maxillofacial Journal 2012;12(Suppl. 8):29.

Chapter 5

Arthroscopic Ankle and Subtalar Arthrodesis – Indications and Surgical Technique

Ricardo Cuéllar, Juan Zaldua, Juan Ponte,
Adrián Cuéllar and Alberto Sánchez

Additional information is available at the end of the chapter

http://dx.doi.org/10.5772/54349

1. Introduction

The history of arthroscopy begins in 1918 when Takagi performed a knee arthroscopy in a cadaver. Due to its narrow joint space, the ankle joint was not considered suitable for arthroscopy in those days. Despite this, in 1939, Takagi described an arthroscopic technique for the ankle joint in a Japanese Orthopaedic Association Journal (Takagi 1939). Watanabe describes in 1972 the anteromedial, anterolateral and posterior portals to the ankle joint. (Watanabe, 1972). In the last few years, thanks to the development of arthroscopic instruments for small joints, and the description of new arthroscopic techniques, ankle and foot arthroscopy have developed significantly (Andrews et al., 1985; Drez et al., 1981; Ferkel, 1996; Gollehon & Drez, 1983; Johnson, 1981; Ogilvie-Harris DJ et al., 1997; Parisien & Vangsness, 1985; Tol & van Dijk, 2004; van Dijk & Scholte, 1997).

Useof m invasive techniques leads to less postoperative pain, lower infection and complication rate and a shorter hospital stay. (Cannon, 2004; Ferkel & Hewitt, 2004; Glick et al., 1996; Golanó et al., 2006; Lui, 2007; Myerson & Quill, 1991).

Degenerative osteoarthritis of the ankle is a common pathology. It is generally associated with traumatic events in the ankle joint, but can also be found in rheumatic patients, infectious processes, osteochondritis, talar necrosis and neurological conditions.

As trauma is the leading cause of this condition it affects younger patients and should be able to ensure a near complete resolution and return to activity.

Arthroscopic instruments and techniques have improved significantly over the last few years, and arthroscopic surgery is now widely used in the ankle joint. It has proven to be a useful tool to diagnose unknown lesions within the arthritic ankle and an efficient therapeutic option to avoid its progression.In our opinion it is a superior alternative to open surgery and it is our first choice technique for both ankle and /or subtalar arthrodesis.

2. Diagnosis of ankle arthritis and preoperative Planning

A complete clinical history and a thorough clinical examination are vital to establish an accurate diagnosis so the correct treatment is indicated. X-rays, CT scan and MRI scan are very useful tools and provide additional information for operative planning.

2.1. Patient assessment

Take into consideration any history of trauma, the nature of the pain, any movements that induce it, whether other joints are involved and record the ankle ROM. Carry out a thorough clinical examination. Consider associated pathologies like rheumatic diseases, gout, diabetes and its relation with Charcot arthropaty or other less common conditions like hemochromatosis.

A complete neurovascular assessment of the limb should be done preoperatively. A note should also be made of the patient´s expectations from the surgery

2.2. Imaging

Weight bearing plain x-rays of the ankle joint provides very useful information. AP, lateral and mortice projections should routinely be taken. A foot X-ray can be very useful to evaluate hind-foot axis and varus /valgus deformities for preoperative planning purposes.

MRI scan is useful to visualize chondral lesions, bone necrosis, and ligamentous injuries.

Technetium Bone Scintigraphy is very helpful to evaluate subtalar joint involvement.

2.3. Surgical indications and contraindications

Ankle, subtalar or double arthrodesis is indicated in cases of painful ankle, subtalar or combined degenerative osteoarthritis, which has not responded to other conservative measures (analgesics, NSAIDs, steroid injections, physiotherapy, and adequate shoe-wear). The most common indications include posttraumatic arthritis, Rheumatoid arthritis, Sero negative arthritis and Charcot´s arthropathy.

The listed contraindications are well known (Table 1). Joint infection, neuropathic conditions and talar necrosis are absolute contraindications.

Axial varus/ valgus deformities >15-20º and anterior tibial shift are relative contraindications. These deformities can be corrected if a wide joint release is associated and is not regarded as a contraindication nowadays.

http://dx.doi.org/10.5772/54349

CONTRAINDICATIONS
ABSOLUTE:
• ACTIVE INFECTION
• ACTIVE CHARCOT ARTHROPATY
• TALAR NECROSIS
• SIGNIFICANT BONE LOSS
• ALGODYSTROPHY
RELATIVE:
• SMOKER
• VARUS/VALGUS "/>15-20º
ANTERIOR TIBIAL SHIFT

Table 1. Ankle arthrodesis contraindications.

3. Method of treatment

In this chapter we intend to describe our method of arthroscopic ankle and subtalar arthrodesis. There are various techniques and their variants described previously in literature. However the basic principles of most remains the same. Majority of the patients are referred to our Arthroscopy Unit with painful arthritic ankles that have not responded to conservative treatment (physiotherapy, NSAIDs). Trauma was the underlying cause leading to painful arthritic joint. A 20 years old female was the youngest patient who underwent the procedure under our care.

In all cases, a diagnostic protocol was completed. This included a complete clinical history, laboratory tests (FBC, ESR, CRP); imaging (X-rays, CT and MRI scans), bone scintigraphy (Tc, Ga); and, occasionally, an ultrasound of the tibialis posterior and Achilles tendons. In some cases bone scintigraphy and CT scans are repeated after a period of 6-12 months to assess subtalar joint involvement.

3.1. Surgical procedure

The anaesthetist determines the appropriate anaesthetic technique: spinal anaesthesia, general anaesthesia or a combination of both. In some cases a popliteal catheter is associated to provide better postoperative pain control.

The patient lies supine on a conventional surgical table in cases of isolated ankle arthrodesis (Figure 1); in prone position if an isolated subtalar arthrodesis is to be done (Figure 2) and in lateral and posterior supine position if both ankle and subtalar arthrodesis are planned (Figure 3).

Joint distraction is required only in a minority of cases (Figure 1).

The procedure tipically lasted between 90 and 100 minutes

3.2. Specific surgical procedures

3.2.1. Ankle arthrodesis

The patient lies in supine position with the affected limb on a leg support in slight abduction. If traction was needed, an external device is attached to the surgeon's waist or a stirrup (Smith and Nephew) is used (Figure 1).

The use of tourniquet and limb axanguination is optional. In our Hospital it is routinely used at the beginning of the arthroscopic procedure and is released after the joint has been reduced and fixed.

The extremity is draped above the knee joint to allow a complete visualization of the leg.

Prior to the incision we recommend identifying and marking the anatomical landmarks of the ankle, specifically: both maleoli, the joint line and the Tibialis Anterior tendon on the medial side, the Peroneus Tertius tendon and the Superficial Peroneal nerve on the lateral side. Superficial Peroneal nerve is palpated like a cord on the lateral aspect of the ankle with the foot in plantar flexion and supination.

Portals: We favour the antero-lateral and the antero-medial arthroscopic portals and follow the standard technique as described by Glick and Morgan. (Glick and Morgan, 1996). After injecting 10-15 cc of saline into the joint, the scope is introduced through the antero-medial portal (medial to the sheath of the Tibialis Anterior tendon, with the ankle in dorsal flexion in order to release the capsule). An incision is made with an nº 15 blade and the capsular incision is dilated with a mosquito. A 30 degree 4,5 mm arthroscope is then introduced into the joint. Using a 21 G needle, the lateral portal is defined. This is located lateral to the Extensor Digitorum tendons and 5 to 10 mm lateral to the Superficial Peroneal Nerve.

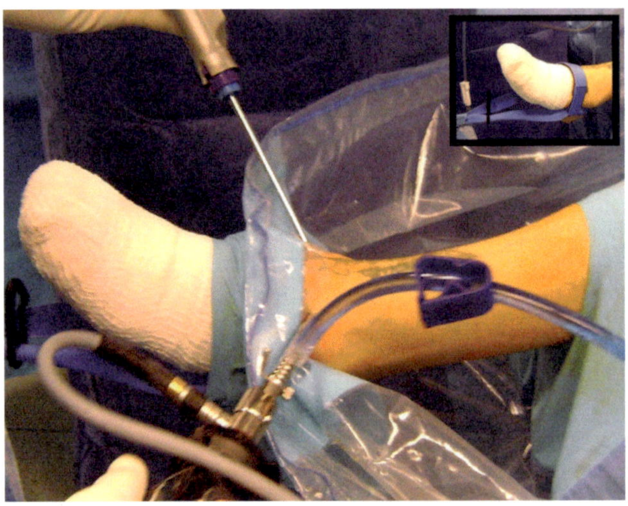

Figure 1. Surgical view of a left ankle arthrodesis in supine position. Triangulation detail and stirrup traction device.

http://dx.doi.org/10.5772/54349

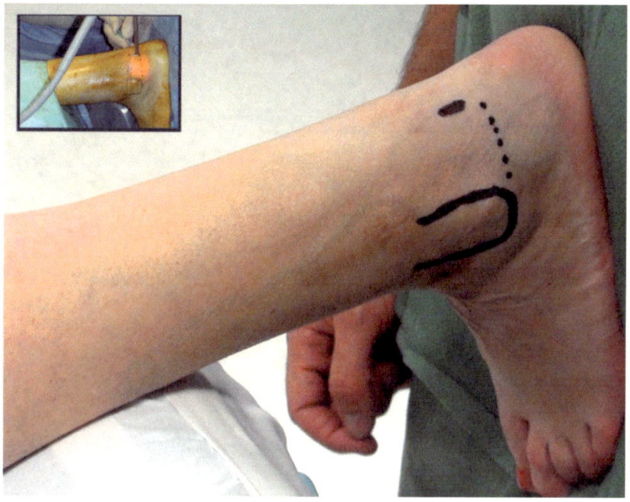

Figure 2. Anatomical landmarks used for left foot subtalar arthrodesis in prone position. Trans-illumination detail.

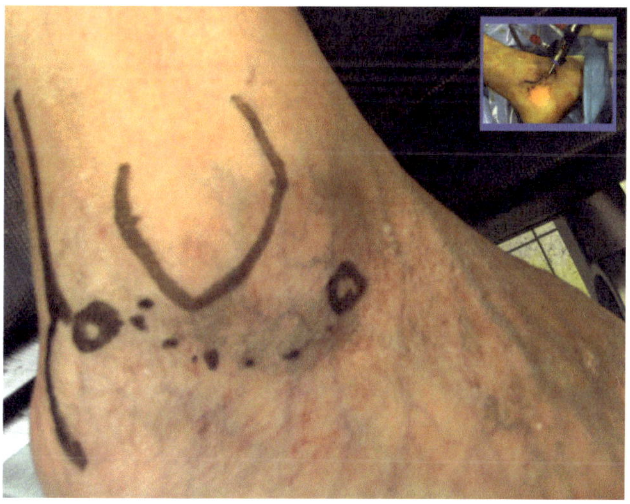

Figure 3. Anatomical landmarks marking before a right ankle and subtalar combined arthrodesis usually done in lateral position. Inset: Use of trans-illumination to define the accessory portal.

Table 2 relates the anterior portals to the ankle joint and the main anatomical structures at risk. Their anatomical relationship is shown in Figure 4.

	Anatomical relations. Anterior approach to the ankle joint	
PORTAL	**RELATIONS**	**STRUCTURES AT RISK**
Anterolateral	Lateral to peroneus tertius tendon	Extensor digitorum Superficial Peroneal Nerve Peroneus Tertius
Anteromedial	Medial to tibialis anterior tendón	Tibialis anterior tendon Extensor hallucis longus Saphenous vein and nerve
Anterior	Between extensor digitorum tendons	Extensor digitorum Dorsalis pedís artery Branches of the superficial and Deep peroneal nerve
Medial Joint line	Between Extensor Hallucis Longus and Tibialis Anterior	Tibialis Anterior tendon Superficial and Deep Peroneal Nerves Dorsalis pedis artery Extensor Hallucis Longus

Table 2. Anatomical relations between the anterior portals to the ankle joint. The main anatomical structures at risk.

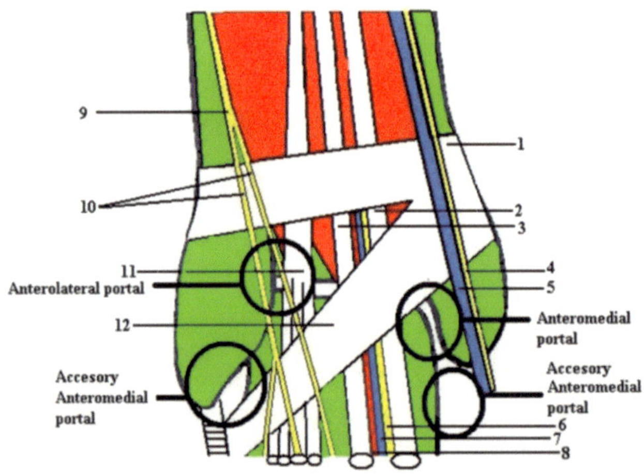

1. Superior Extensor Retinaculum, 2. Tibialis Anterior, 3. Extensor Hallucis Longus, 4. Saphenous Nerve, 5. Saphenous Vein, 6. Deep Peroneal Nerve, 7. Dorsalis Pedis Vein, 8. Dorsalis Pedis Artery, 9. Superficial Peroneal Nerve, 10. Superficial branches of th Superficial Peroneal Nerve, 11. Extensor Digitorum Longus, 12. Inferior Flexor Retinaculum

Figure 4. Illustration showing the anterior arthroscopic portals to the ankle joint and their anatomical relations with surrounding structures (Right ankle, anterior view).

The soft tissues are then debrided with a powered blade at 10.000 rpm. Once the articular surface is visualized, we proceed to shave it with a curette or with a 4mm powered bur. A small retractor can be used to better visualize the posterior joint and the lateral gutters (Figure 5). As the bone is being removed, access becomes easier and traction can be released.

http://dx.doi.org/10.5772/54349

3.2.1.1. Correction of severe deformities

We strongly recommend a thorough debridement of the lateral gutters. This allows a good view of the capsular insertions (Figure 6).

In cases of severe valgus /varus deformities, the capsule should be widely released to allow free mobilization and opposition of the joint surfaces in order to achieve a correct anatomical alignment. Figure 7 shows a case of severe deformity where the anterior tibial shift is corrected.

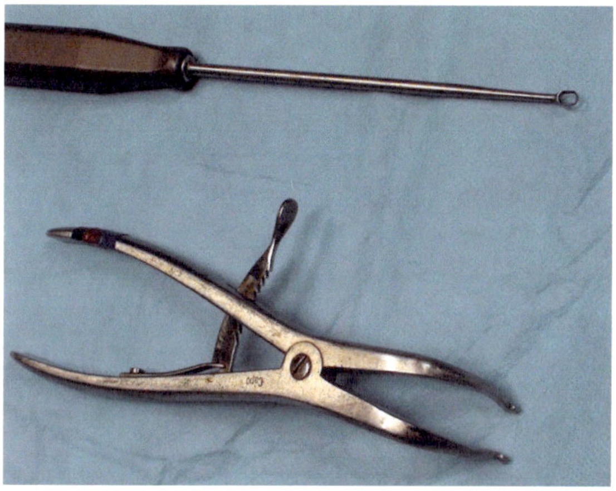

Figure 5. Surgical instruments needed. Different sized curettes and a small bivalved retractor that can be introduced through an extended arthroscopic portal.

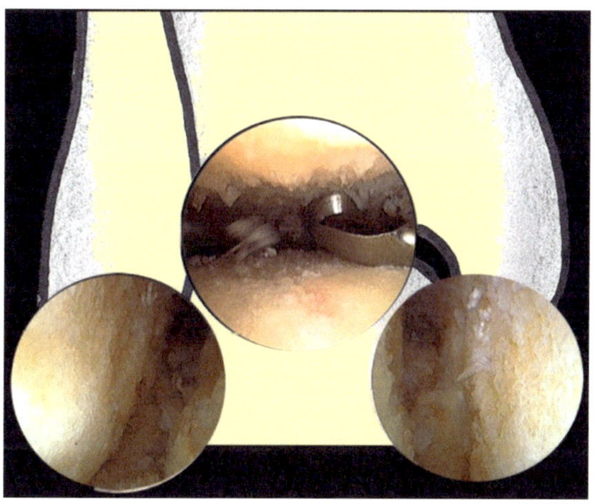

Figure 6. Photo composition of an ankle arthrodesis. Several aspects of the surgical debridement and release of the gutters in order to visualize the capsular insertion that has to be resected in cases of severe deformity.

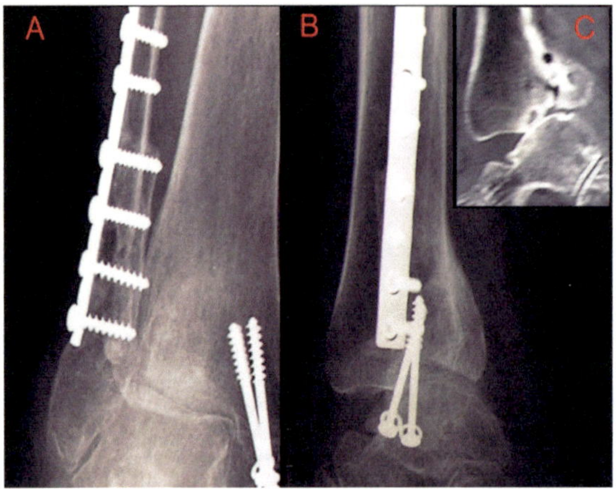

Figure 7. Gross ankle deformity (anterior tibial shift) following an old fracture dislocation of the ankle that had been operated in the past. AP and lateral X-rays.- CT scan detail.

If the articular surfaces were sclerotic, perforations should be made to create a bleeding bed. Exceptionally, a bone graft may be needed to fill bone defects and achieve a better joint congruency (Figure 8).

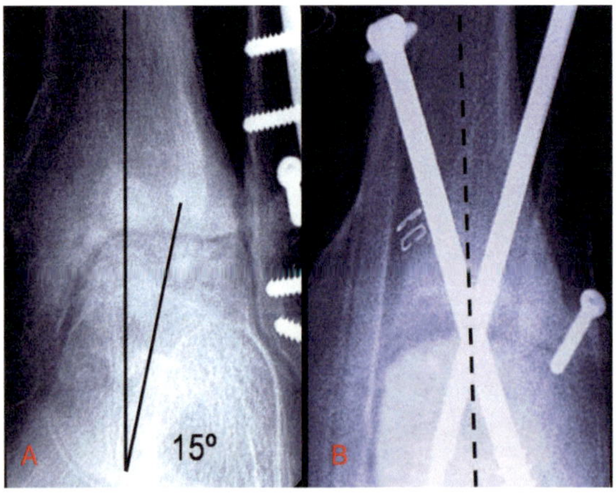

Figure 8. AP X-ray showing severe axial deformity in 15º of varus in an old fracture dislocation of a right ankle that had been operated in the past. Right. Intraoperative control previous to the introduction of the second screw. Notice the axial correction and the placement of a bone graft in the medial side to improve joint congruency.

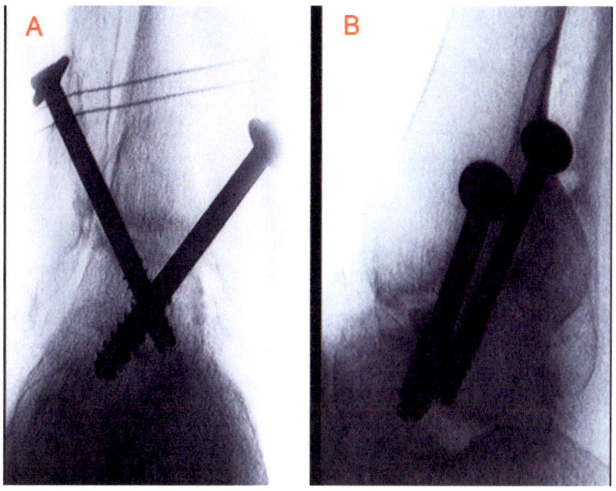

Figure 9. Intraoperative AP and lateral X-ray control showing correction of the anterior tibial shift of figure 7 case.

3.2.1.2. Correction control

Visual and radiological checks of the ankle axis are done with the leg in extension after debriding the articular surfaces and before inserting the screws (Figures 8, 9).

The ankle should be fixed in neutral dorsiflexion, 0-5º of valgus, 5-10º of external rotation (or similar to the contralateral ankle) with a slight posterior talar tilt. Shortening should be avoided or kept to a minimum

3.2.1.3. Fixation

Once the joint surfaces are congruent and the axis of the ankle joint is correct, 2 Kirschner wires are introduced as described by Glick and Morgan (Glick and Morgan, 1996). The first wire is introduced anterolateraly 5 cm above the joint line. It should be angled 10-20 º to target the posterior half of the talus. Care should be taken not to damage the Sural Nerve or the Peroneus Superficialis tendon.

The second wire is introduced postero-medialy and anterior to the Tibialis Posterior tendon.

In order to improve stability, it should be directed in an X-crossed shape from the postero-medial aspect of the tibia towards the antero-central area of the talar dome (Figure 10).

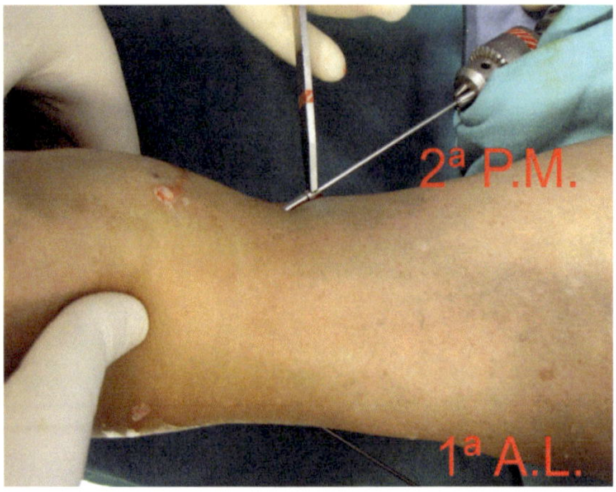

Figure 10. X-ray guided ankle arthrodesis fixation with 2 Kirschner wires. The first one introduced anteromedialy 5 cm above the joint line, angled 10-20º posteriorly. The second wire posteromedialy and directed anterior to the Tibialis Anterior sheath.

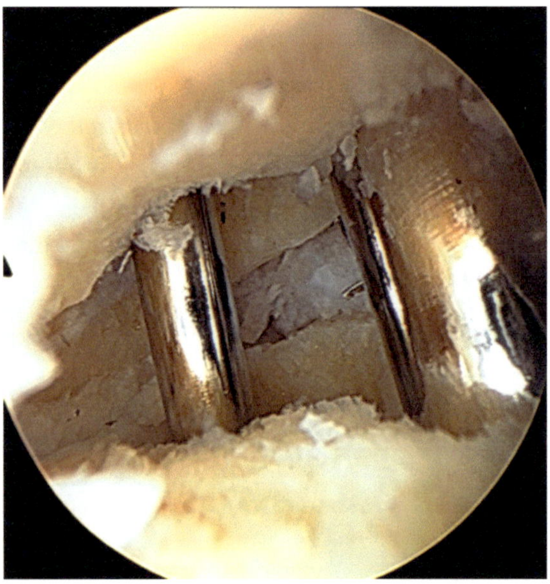

Figure 11. Arthroscopic control to assess the guide wires is correctly positioned to avoid screw contact.

http://dx.doi.org/10.5772/54349

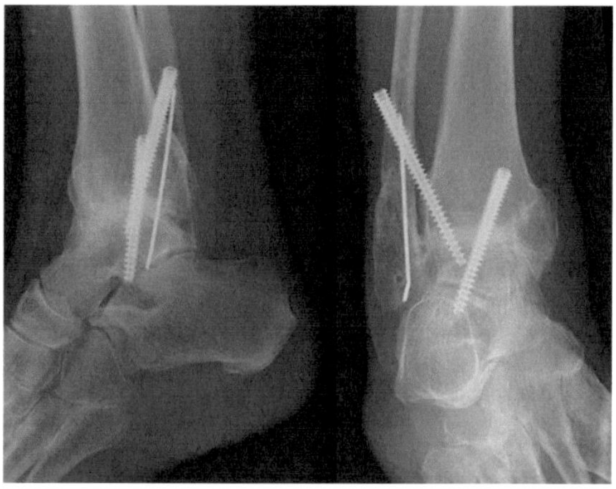

Figure 12. X-ray showing consolidation of an ankle arthrodesis despite screw interposition.

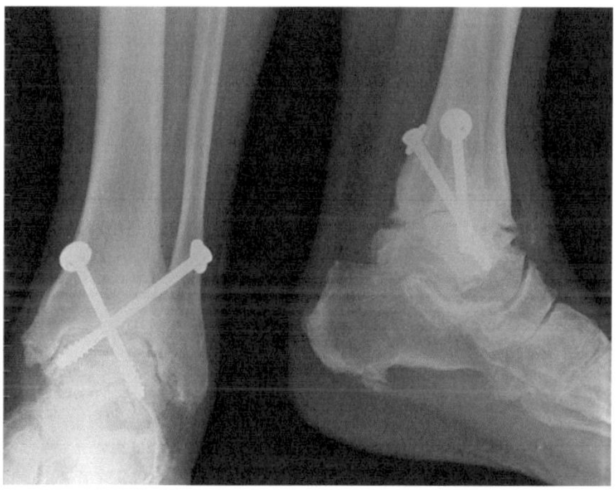

Figure 13. Delayed consolidation 6 months after ankle arthrodesis. Using 6,5 mm conventional cannulated screws.

We recommend visualizing the guide wires position through the arthroscope to avoid the screws interfering with each other (Figure 11). In the case shown in Figure 12, the lateral screw got blocked with the medial one. Despite our efforts to introduce it further or to withdraw the screw, this was not possible. The screw was left and the arthrodesis consolidated successfully.

Definitive fixation is achieved with 2 cannulated screws creating compression independently as described by Glick and Morgan. (Glik and Morgan, 1996). Originally we used 6,5 mm screws, but after having a few cases of delayed consolidation (Figure 13), we now use Acutrak (Acumed®), size 6/7 screws.

At the end of the procedure, AP and lateral X-rays should be taken (Figure 9).

3.2.1.4. *Postoperative protocol*

The leg is immobilized in a well padded plaster backslab that is removed after two weeks together with the stitches. A plaster boot is then applied allowing partial weight bearing. Some studies allow full weight bearing after 2 weeks (Cannon, 2004).

Control X-rays are taken at 6-8 weeks to assess bone consolidation.

If the X-rays are not conclusive, a CT scan may be useful.

At 10 weeks free full weight bearing is allowed.

A course of 4 to 4 weeks of Physiotherapy may be beneficial to gain propioception, particularly in older patients.

It is recommended to use MBT shoes.

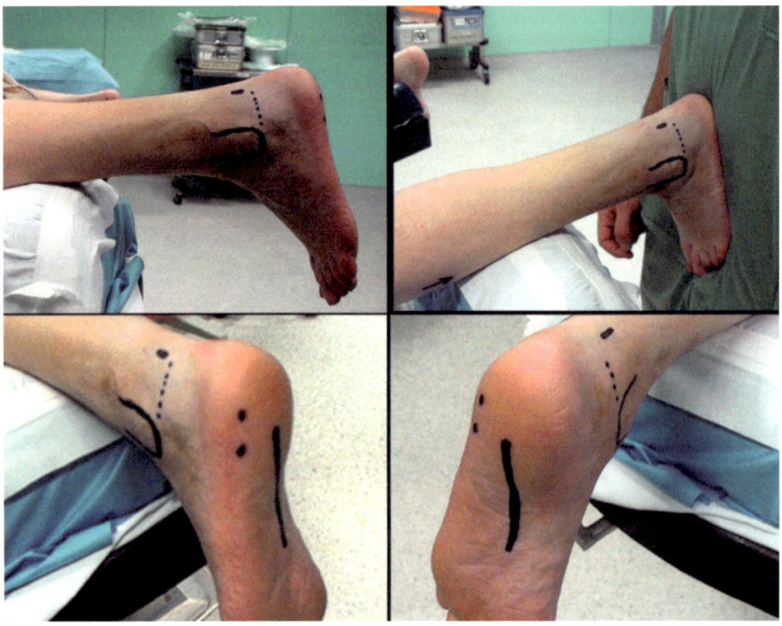

Figure 14. Photo composition of a subtalar arthrodesis of a left ankle. The patient lies prone with the ankle out of the table resting on a roll. The contralateral leg is positioned in abduction. The anatomical landmarks are highlighted. Both malleoli, the Achilles Tendon and the axis of the first ray are marked.

3.2.2. *Subtalar arthrodesis*

The posterior arthroscopic ankle approach was described as subtalar approach in 1985 by Parisien and Vangness. (Parisien & Vangsness, 1985). In 2000 Van Dijk described the two posterior ankle portals (van Dijk et al., 2000; van Dijk, 2006). Pérez- Carro sugested the subtalar approach with the patient set in prone position (Pérez-Carro et al., 2007).

http://dx.doi.org/10.5772/54349

The patient is positioned prone with one third of the ankle set off the table. This rests on a sand roll so the ankle is elevated in order to allow dorsiflexion and better access to the subtalar joint. The contralateral leg is kept in abduction (Figure 14).

Both maleoli and the Achilles tendon are marked with a pen. An incision is made just above the medial maleolus 3mm medial to the Achilles tendon. After dilating the portal with a mosquito, a 4, 5 mm arthroscope is introduced with a 30º lens, directed towards the first space (Figure 15).

With the arthroscope resting on bone, the antero medial portal is made. We use the touch and slide technique to get oriented with the motorized cutter (Figure 16).

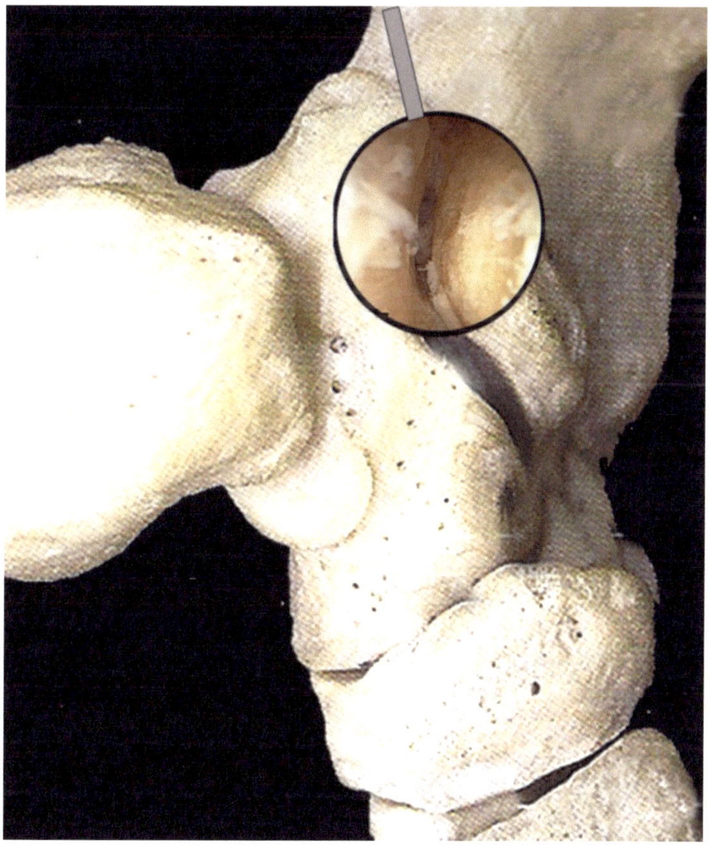

Figure 15. An incision is made lateral to the Achilles T and the arthroscope is introduced towards the 1st space.

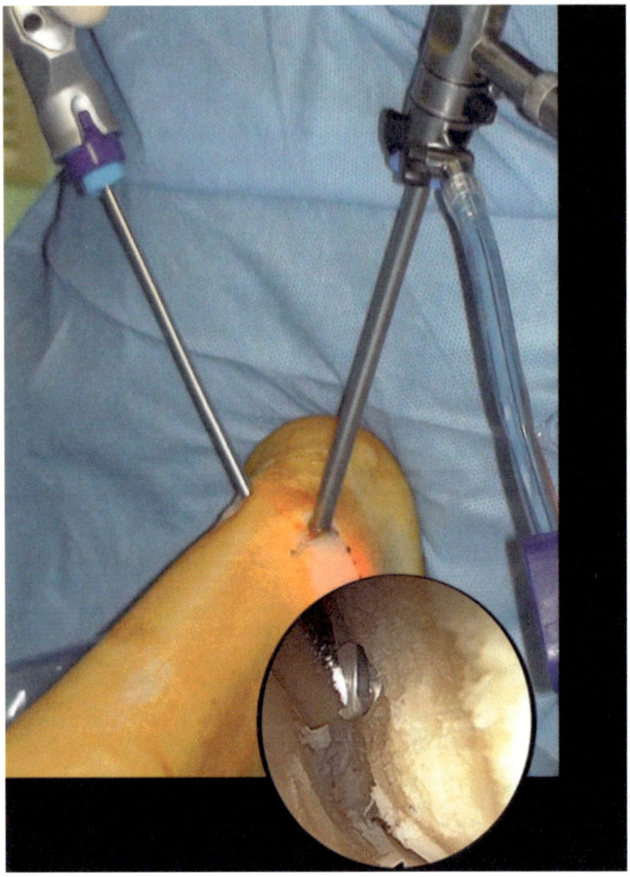

Figure 16. Orientation technique resting the shaver on top of the arthroscope and sliding it until visual contact is made.

Anatomical relations. Posterior approach to the ankle joint		
PORTAL	**RELATIONS**	**STRUCTURES AT RISK**
POSTEROLATERAL	Lateral to the Achilles tendon	Sural Nerve Lesser saphenous vein
POSTEROMEDIAL	Medial to the Achilles Tendon	Tibialis Posterior artery Tibial nerve and Calcaneal branches Flexor hallucis longus tendon Flexor digitorum longus

Table 3. Anatomical relations between the posterior portals to the ankle joint and the main anatomical structures at risk.

Table 3 relates the anterior portals to the ankle joint and the main anatomical structures at risk. Their anatomical relationship is shown in Figure 17

http://dx.doi.org/10.5772/54349

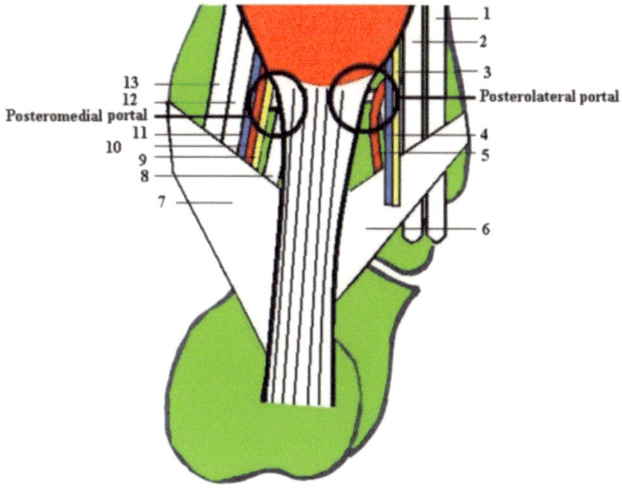

1. Peroneus Longus, 2. Peroneus Brevis, 3. Sural Nerve, 4. Lesser Saphenous Vein, 5. Peroneal Artery, 6. Peroneal Retinaculum, 7. Flexor Retinaculum, 8. Flexor Hallucius Longus, 9. Tibialis Posterior Nerve, 10. Tibialis Posterior Artery, 11. Tibialis Posterior Vein, 12. Flexor Digitorum Longus, 13. Tibialis Posterior

Figure 17. Illustration showing the posterior arthroscopic portals to the ankle joint and their anatomical relations (Right ankle, posterior view).

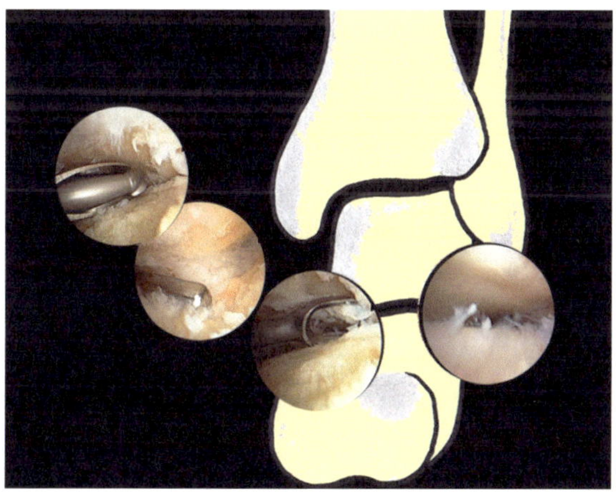

Figure 18. Photo composition of a subtalar arthrodesis. Initial visualization and arthroscopic debridement.

The Flexor Hallucis Longus tendon should be identified. The neurovascular bundle lies medial to it. If the tendon is found to be compressed either by osteophytes or by soft tissue adhesions, the flexor retinaculum should be released and a synovectomy should be carried out.

The soft tissues are debrided with a powered synovial blade at 1200 rpm until the subtalar joint space is well defined. The articular surfaces are then roughened with curettes or a motorized 4 mm burr until the posterior facet of the talus is well visualized (Figure 18).

With a lateral ankle x-ray, the subtalar articular surfaces and the hindfoot position are checked before proceeding with the fixation.

Figure 19 shows the surgical field during a subtalar arthrodesis.

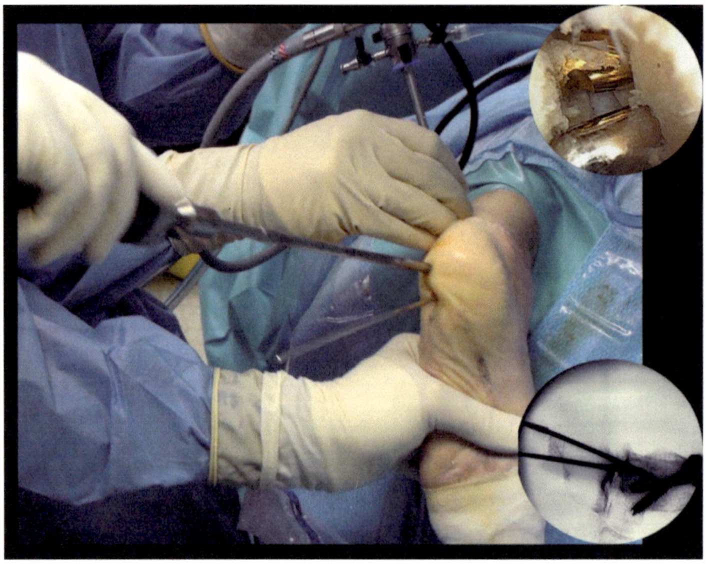

Figure 19. Subtalar arthrodesis of a left foot in prone position. Arthroscopic control (right upper corner). X-ray control (right inferior corner).

3.2.2.1. Correction control

Visual and radiological checks of the ankle axis should be carried out with the joint at 90º flexion during the procedure and before completing the screw insertion

3.2.2.2. Fixation

2 temporary Kirschner wires are introduced in neutral position from the postero-medial aspect of the calcaneum. A check X-ray should be taken. If the position is satisfactory, we proceed with the fixation using two size 6/7 Acutrak (Acumed) cannulated screws (Figure 20).

3.2.2.3. Postoperative recommendations

A compressive bandage is applied and early ankle movements are encouraged.

During the first 6 weeks partial weight bearing is allowed in a Walker type orthosis.

Full weight bearing is allowed when X-rays show the posterior facets are consolidated and the patient is pain free.

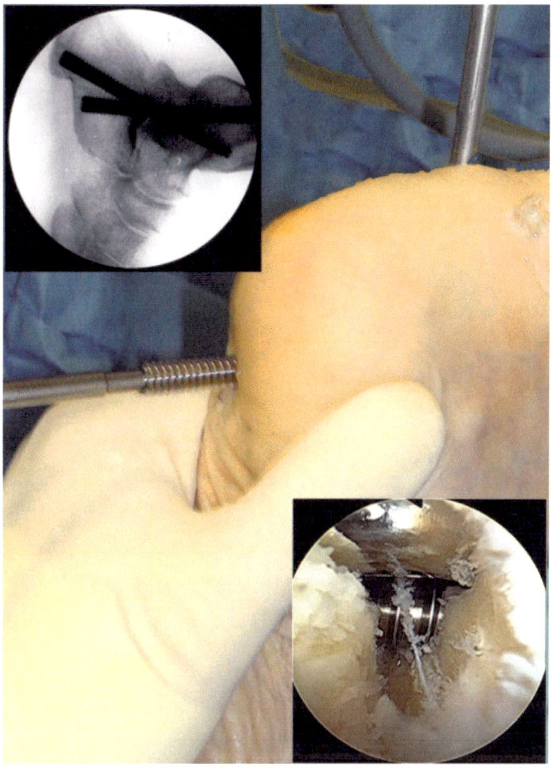

Figure 20. Screw insertion of subtalar arthrodesis of a left foot in prone position: X-ray control (left upper corner); arthroscopic control (right inferior corner).

3.2.3. Combined ankle and subtalar arthrodesis

Combined ankle and subtalar arthrodesis can be done focusing on each separate joint at a time during the same surgical procedure (Lui, 2007). In this case, the patient is initially positioned prone (Figure 3), and is then changed to the lateral position (Figure 21).

The use of the tibio-talo-calcaneal nail (Boer et al., 2007; Gagneux et al., 1997; Hammett et al., 2005; Jehan et al., 2011; Mendicino et al., 2004; Pelton et al., 2006) allows approaching the subtalar joint through an extended lateral approach over the sinus tarsi (Figure 3) using the lateral portals as described by Parisien (Parisien & Vangsness, 1985).

The approach to the ankle and to the subtalar joint can be done either arthroscopicaly or via a mini opening assisted with X-ray control. In both cases the patient is initially positioned prone and then changed to the lateral position when approaching the susbtalar joint.

In some cases, i.e. rheumatoid patients, where no major axial corrections need to be made and the joints are severely affected, the reaming done during the intramedulary nailing procedure may provide enough bone graft and burring the subtalar joint may not be needed.

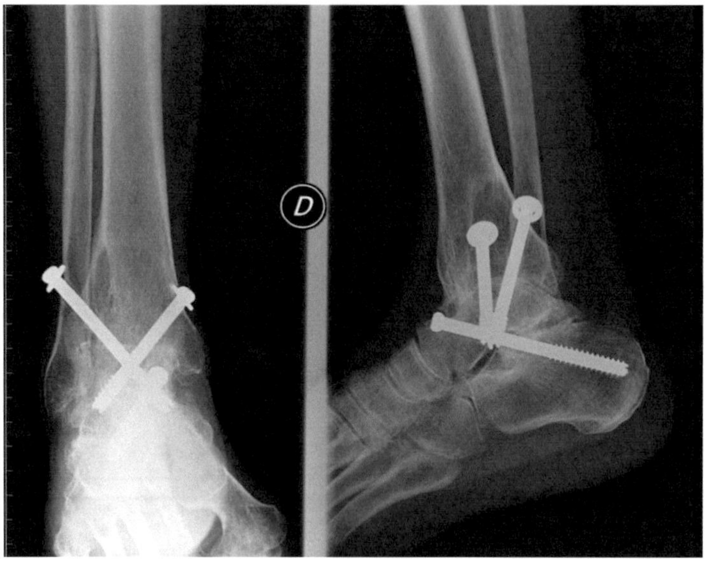

Figure 21. X-ray showing consolidated ankle and subtalar arthrodesis that were done separately.

3.2.3.1. Surgical recommendations

In cases of tibio-talo-calcaneal arthrodesis, we use the Trigen HFN (hind foot nail), Smith & Nephew (Figure 22). This offers the possibility of introducing longitudinally an extra screw incorporating the calcaneocuboid joint.

The most important step in this technique is positioning of the guide wire in the centre of the tibia. The entry point in the plantar aspect of the foot should rather be more medial than lateral and should be assisted with X- ray control. If the position of the guide wire is not correct, a second guide wire can be introduced through the additional holes provided in the entry positioning tool.

Relevant points for a correct indication and successful surgery are summarized in Table 4.

4. Clinical evidence

We have revised retrospectively 62 cases of ankle arthrodesis operated between 1997 and 2007 in our University Hospital. 50 cases were done by conventional open surgery and the remaining 12 were done arthroscopically.

Ankle arthroscopy offers a lower morbidity and infection rate. It provides a much better visualization and access to the lateral gutters, which allows a wider capsular release that facilitates mobilization of the joint surfaces in cases of severe axial deformities or anterior tibial shift.

http://dx.doi.org/10.5772/54349

TIPS FOR THE SURGERY
• Diagnostic Local anesthetic injections in the tibial and subtalar joint to identify the source of pain
• Rule out a fixed hindfoot deformity that may need a different type of surgery
• Beware of the Superficial peroneal Nerve laterally
• The patient position should allow good access to the Image Intensifier
• Check hindfoot alignment following the provisional fixation
• Use the "touch and slide technique" to get oriented
• Have both straight and curved curettes available
• Once the bone surfaces are roughened, release the tourniquet so a bleeding bed can be visualized
• Visualize the guide wires position through the arthroscope to avoid the screws interfering
• Both screws should be mechanically independent

Table 4. Relevant points for a correct indication and successful surgery

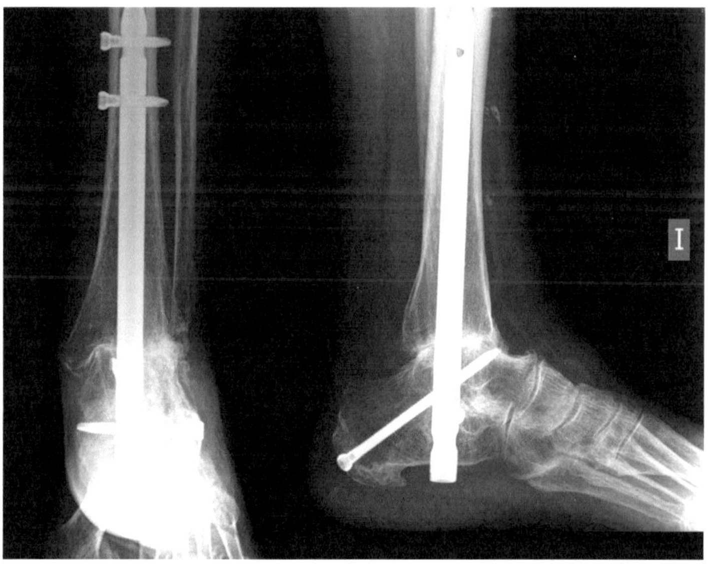

Figure 22. X-ray showing a combined ankle and subtalar arthrodesis by intramedullary nailing.

Traditionally, major varus/valgus deformities >15º or anterior tibial shift were regarded as absolute contraindications for this technique. In the last few years this technique is routinely used in our Hospital environment even in cases of major ankle deformities (Figure 23). These advantages are summarized in Table 5.

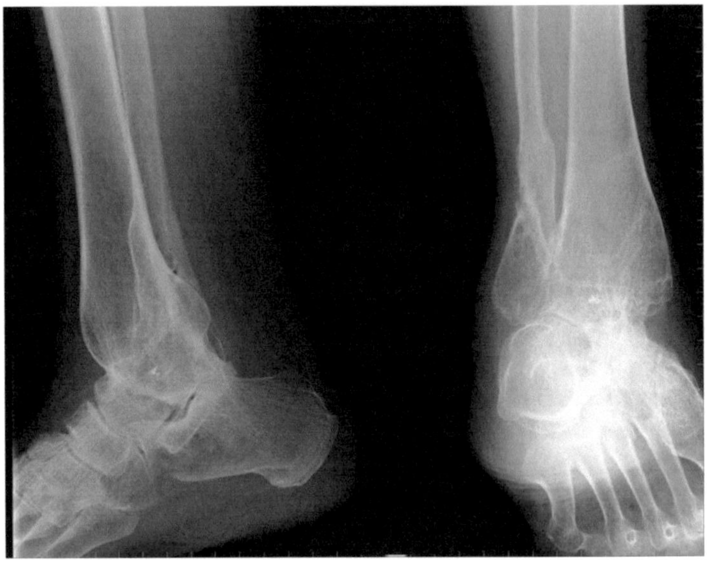

Figure 23. year follow up control X-ray showing radiological consolidation. Note the correction of the anterior tibial shift in AP and lateral views compared to figures 7 and 9.

Features	Advantages
Better pathology visualization Better access to lateral gutters	Allows treatment of severe axial "/>15º and anterior tibial shift deformities
Less surgical Trauma Less damage to bone vascularization	Less postoperative morbidity Lower complication rate Shorter hospital stay
Better access to associated pathology No alteration of bone contours	Allows double / triple arthrodesis

Table 5. Features and main advantages of arthroscopic versus open ankle arthrodesis

There is no significant difference between the mean consolidation times with either technique (4 to 6 months). There were a few cases of delayed consolidation in patients were conventional cannulated screws were used (Figure 13). Despite this, all cases consolidated successfully.

Subtalar ostoarthritis developed following arthroscopic ankle arthrodesis in one case and following traditional open surgery in another case. There were no signs of subtalar arthritis in the pre-op Xrays or bone scintigraphy- in neither case and diagnostic injections with local anesthetic did rule out subtalar involvement. Osteoarthritis developed 24 months following surgery and both cases required subsequent subtalar arthrodesis (Figure 24).

In a nail subtalar joint arthrodesis It would appear reasonable to assume that both articular surfaces should be roughened but is no clinical evidence that the consolidation rate is higher than in cases that have not been burred.

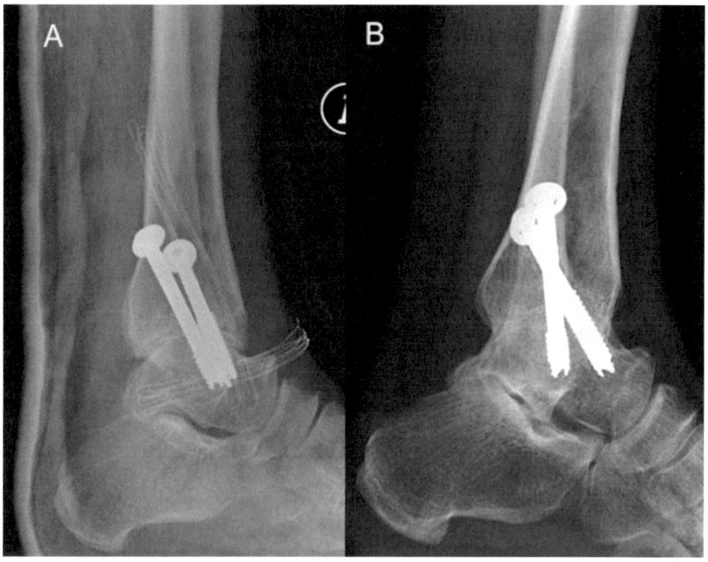

Figure 24. Subtalar osteoartritis 27 months following ankle arthrodesis.

5. Discussion

Arthroscopic ankle arthrodesis allows joint fixation maintaining the main joint anatomy and keeping subcondral bone loss to a minimum.

The complication rate in the inmediate postoperative period is smaller compared to open surgery. The convalescence time is shorter. Myerson & Quill, 1991).

The operating time and the hospital stay are shorter. (O´Brien et al., 1999).

The infection rate and other soft tissue complications rate is lower in arthroscopically treated cases

The bone consolidation rate is similar in both groups. In our experience 85% of ankle arthrodesis had consolidated after 4-5 months postop.

Recent studies have shown good or excellent results in 85 of cases with a low complication and non-union rate (Glick et al., 1996; Tasto et al., 2000; Wasserman et al., 2004; Zvijac et al., 2002).

In severe varus/valgus deformities>10º with anterior tibial shift, a good correction can be achieved arthroscopically if an adequate capsular joint release is made. This was regarded as a contraindication in the past.

This technique allows early postoperative mobilization and is ideal in elder patients with associated inflammatory processes.

Excellent results have been published in some series of subtalar arthroscopic arthrodesis, where the consolidation time was 8, 9 weeks with no infection or non union cases reported.

Ankle arthroscopy is constantly developing and has become the favourite surgical technique amongst many ankle and foot surgeons.

6. Conclusions

Arthroscopic ankle arthrodesis is a reproductible and reliable, technique with a lower complication rate than traditional open ankle surgery.

It is a rapidly developing technique that broadens the possibilities and the indications of ankle and foot surgery.

The long term results are similar to those of traditional open ankle surgery.

Arthroscopic ankle and subtalar arthrodesis induces less trauma to the soft tisues and this translates in a lower complication rate, a shorter hospital stay, an early mobilization and a higher success rate. All these factors have made arthroscopic surgery, our first choice technique for ankle and subtalar arthrodesis.

Author details

Ricardo Cuéllar[1], Juan Zaldua[1], Juan Ponte[2], Adrián Cuéllar[3] and Alberto Sánchez[3]

1 University Hospital Donostia (San Sebastián), Spain

2 Policlinica Gipuzkoa (San Sebastián), Spain

3 Galdakao Unansolo Hospital (Galdakao), Spain

References

[1] Andrews, J. R, Previte, W. J, & Carson, W. G. (1985). Arthroscopy of the ankle: Technique and normal anatomy. Foot & Ankle, PMID 4043889., 6, 29-33.

[2] Boer, R, Mader, K, Pennig, D, & Verheyen, C. C. (2007). Tibiotalocalcaneal arthrodesis using a reamed retrograde locking nail. Clinical Orthopaedics and Related Research, 0000-9921X.(463), 151-156.

[3] Cannon, L. (2004). Early weight bearing is safe following arthroscopic ankle arthrodesis. The Journal of Foot & Ankle Surgery, 1268-7731, 10, 135-139.

[4] Drez, D. Jr.; Guhl, J.H. & Gollehon, D.L. ((1981). Ankle arthroscopy: Technique and indications. The Journal of Foot & Ankle Surgery, PMID 7341387., 2, 138-143.

[5] Ferkel, R. D. (1996). Arthroscopic Surgery: In: The Foot and Ankle. Philadelphia, Lippincott-Raven (1996). 100397510934

[6] Ferkel, R. D, & Hewitt, M. (2004). Long-term results of arthroscopic ankle arthrodesis. Foot & Ankle International Journal., 1071-1007, 26, 275-280.

[7] Gagneux, E, Gerard, F, Garbuio, P, & Vichard, P. (1997). Treatment of complex fractures of the ankle and their sequellae using trans-plantar intramedullary nailing. Acta Orthopaedica Belga, Nº 4, (1997), PMID 9479784., 63, 294-304.

[8] Glick, J. M, Morgan, C. D, Myerson, M. S, Sampson, T. G, & Mann, J. A. (1996). Ankle arthrodesis using an arthroscopic method: long term follow up of 34 cases. The Journal of Arthroscopy and Related Surgery, Nº 8, (1996), 0749-8063, 12, 428-434.

[9] Golanó, P, Vega, J, Pérez-carro, L, & Götzens, V. (2006). Ankle anatomy for the arthroscopist. Part I: The portals. The Orthopedic Clinics of North America, PMID 1570142., 11, 275-296.

[10] Gollehon, D. L, & Drez, D. (1983). Ankle artroscopy approaches and technique. Orthopedics ISSNN 1590-9921., 6, 1150-1158.

[11] Hammett, R, Hepple, S, Forster, B, & Winson, I. (2005). Tibiotalocalcaneal (hindfoot) arthrodesis by retrograde intramedullary nailing using a curved locking nail. The results of 52 procedures. Foot & Ankle International Journal, 1071-1007, 27, 810-815.

[12] Jehan, S, Shakeel, M, Bing, A. J, & Hill, S. O. (2011). The success of tibiotalocalcaneal arthrodesis with intramedullary nailing--a systematic review of the literature. Acta Orthopaedica Belga, Nº 5, (2011), PMID 22187841., 77, 644-651.

[13] Johnson, L. L. (1981). Ankle arthroscopy In: Diagnostic and Surgical Arthroscopy. St Louis, Mosby-Year Book (1981), 0-80162-535-1, 412-419.

[14] Lui, T. H. Arthroscopy and endoscopy ot the foot and ankle: Indications for new techniques. The Journal of Arthroscopy and Related Surgery, Nº 8, ((2007). 0749-8063, 23, 889-902.

[15] Mendicino, R. W, Catanzariti, A. R, Saltrick, K. R, Dombek, M. F, Tullis, B. L, Statler, T. K, & Johnson, B. M. (2004). Tibiotalocalcaneal arthrodesis with retrograde intramedullary mailing. The Journal of Foot & Ankle Surgery, PMID 15057853., 43(2), 83-86.

[16] Myerson, M. S, & Quill, G. (1991). Ankle arthrodesis. A comparison of an arthroscopic and an open method of treatment. Clinical Orthopaedics and Related Research, 0000-9921X.(268), 84-95.

[17] Brien, O, Hart, T. S, Shereff, T. S, Stone, M. J, & Jhonson, J. J. ((1999). Open versus arthroscopic ankle arthrodesis: a comparative study. Foot & Ankle International Journal, PMID 10395339., 20, 368-374.

[18] Ogilvie-harris, D. J, Gilbart, M. K, & Chorney, K. (1997). Chronic pain following ankle sprains in athletes: The role of arthroscopic surgery. The Journal of Arthroscopy and Related Surgery, Nº 5, (1997), 0749-8063, 13, 564-574.

[19] Parisien, J. S, & Vangsness, T. (1985). Arthroscopy of the subtalar joint: An experimental approach. The Journal of Arthroscopy and Related Surgery, Nº 1, (1985), 0749-8063, 1, 53-57.

[20] Parisien, J. S, & Vangsness, T. (1985). Operative arthroscopy of the ankle: three years ′experience. Clinical Orthopedics and Related Reserch 0000-9921X., 199, 46-53.

[21] Pelton, K, Hofer, J. K, & Thordarson, D. B. (2006). Tibiotalocalcaneal arthrodesis using a dynamically locked retrograde intramedullary nail. Foot & Ankle International Journal, Nº 10, (2004), PMID 17054874., 27, 759-763.

[22] Pérez-carro, L. Golanó, P & Vega, J. ((2007). Arthroscopic subtalar arthrodesis: The posterior approach in prone position. The Journal of Arthroscopy and Related Surgery, Nº 4, (2007), e1-445.e4), 0749-8063, 23, 445.

[23] Takagi, K. (1939). The classic. Arthroscope. Kengi Takagi. Journal Japanesse Orthopedic Association. Clinical Orthopedics and Related Reserch 0000-9921X., 167, 6-8.

[24] Tasto, J. P. (1999). Arthroscopic subtalar arthrodesis. Presented at the Annual Meeting of the American Academy of Orthopaedic Surgeons, Anaheim, California, February , 4-8.

[25] Tasto, J. P, Frey, C, Laimans, P, et al. (2000). Arthroscopic ankle arthrodesis. American Academy of Orthopaedic Surgeosns, Instructional Course Lectures, PMID 16985465., 49, 259-280.

[26] Tol, J. L, & Van Dijk, C. N. (2004). Etiology of the anterior ankle impigment syndrome: A descriptive anatomical study. Foot & Ankle International Journal, Nº 6, (2004), 1071-1007, 25, 382-386.

[27] Van Dijk, C. N, & Scholte, D. (1997). Arthroscopy of the ankle joint. The Journal of Arthroscopy and Related Surgery, Nº 1, (1997), 0749-8063, 13, 90-96.

[28] Van Dijk, C. N, Scholten, P. E, & Krips, R. (2000). A 2-portal endoscopic approach for diagnosis and treatment of posterior ankle pathology. The Journal of Arthroscopy and Related Surgery, Nº 8, (2000), 0749-8063, 16, 871-876.

[29] Van Dijk, C. N. (2006). Hind-foot endoscopy for posterior ankle pain. American Academy of Orthopaedic Surgeons, Instructional Course Lecture, PMID 16958469., 55, 545-554.

[30] Wasserman, L. R, Saltzman, C. L, & Amendola, A. (2004). Minimally invasive ankle reconstruction: Current scope and indications. The Orthopedics Clinics of the North America, ISNN, 35(2), 247-253.

[31] Watanabe, M. (1972). Selfoc-Arthroscope (Watanabe arthroscope). Monograph. Tokyo: Teishin Hospital, 1972.(24)

[32] Zvijac, J. E, Lemak, L, Schurhoff, M. R, Hechtman, K. S, & Uribe, J. W. (2002). Analysis of arthroscopically assisted ankle arthrodesis. The Journal of Arthroscopy and Related Surgery, 0749-8063, 18(1), 70-75.

Chapter 6

Subtalar Arthroscopy and a Technical Note on Arthroscopic Interosseous Talocalcaneal Ligament Reconstruction

Jiao Chen, Hu Yuelin and Guo Qinwei

Additional information is available at the end of the chapter

http://dx.doi.org/10.5772/55112

1. Introduction

1.1. History of subtalar arthroscopy

The history of arthroscopy can be traced back to 1912 when the Danish physician Severin Nordentoft reported on arthroscopies of the knee joint at the Proceedings of the 4lst Congress of the German Society of Surgeons at Berlin [1]. Till seventy three years later was the first article on subtalar arthroscopy published in which Parisien did a cadaver study and introduced the arthroscopic approaches in detail[2]. Frey C compared three portals of subtalar arthroscopy on visualization area and safety in an article published in 1994[3]. Lundeen described ankle and subtalar joint fusion under arthroscopy in the same year[4]. Afterwards, as the advance of surgical technique many diseases can be treated under subtalar arthroscopy. However, to observe all structures in subtalar joint is still not easy and more efforts should be made to improve the subtalar arthroscopy technique.

2. Anatomy of subtalar joint

The subtalar joint is comprised of two articulations: anterior subtalar joint and posterior subtalar joint divide by the sinus tarsi and tarsal canal. The anterior subtalar joint is formed by posterior facet of the navicular, convex head of the talus, oval and slightly convex middle talar facet, anterior and middle facets of the superior surface of os calcis. The floor of the joint is formed by the plantar surface of the talar head with the dorsal surface of the spring ligament. This articulation is also called the talocalcaneonavicular joint[5]. The posterior subtalar joint is posterior talocalcaneal joint consisting of the inferior posterior facet of the talus and the superior posterior facet of the calcaneus, the axis of which runs obliquely forwards, downwards and outwards. The subtalar joint produces movement of supination which is composed of plantarflexion in the parasagittal plane, inversion in the frontal plane, and adduction in the transverse plane and pronation which is composed of eversion in the frontal plane, abduction in the transverse plane, and dorsiflexion in the parasagittal plane[6,7].

Between anterior and posterior subtalar articulations lies the sinus tarsi laterally and tarsal canal medially. Two separate groups of ligament structures lie in the sinus tarsi and tarsal canal. The lateral group of ligament structures in sinus tarsi includes lateral and intermedial root of the inferior extensor retinaculum. The medial group of ligament structures in tarsal canal consists of medial root of the inferior extensor retinaculum, cervical ligament and interosseous talocalcaneal ligament (ITCL). The ITCL originates from the sinus calcanei, orients proximally and medially and inserts into the sulcus of the talus. It is composed of two bands. The anterior band orients in an oblique direction from the sinus calcanei anteriorly to the inferior talar neck while the posterior band attached to the posterior sinus tali. This ligament contributes to the subtalar supination stability[5]. The cervical ligament inserts on the calcaneus anterior to the posterior talocalcaneal joint, goes posteromedially and ends on the talar external border of the tarsal canal. It also contributes to the subtalar stability. (Figure 1)

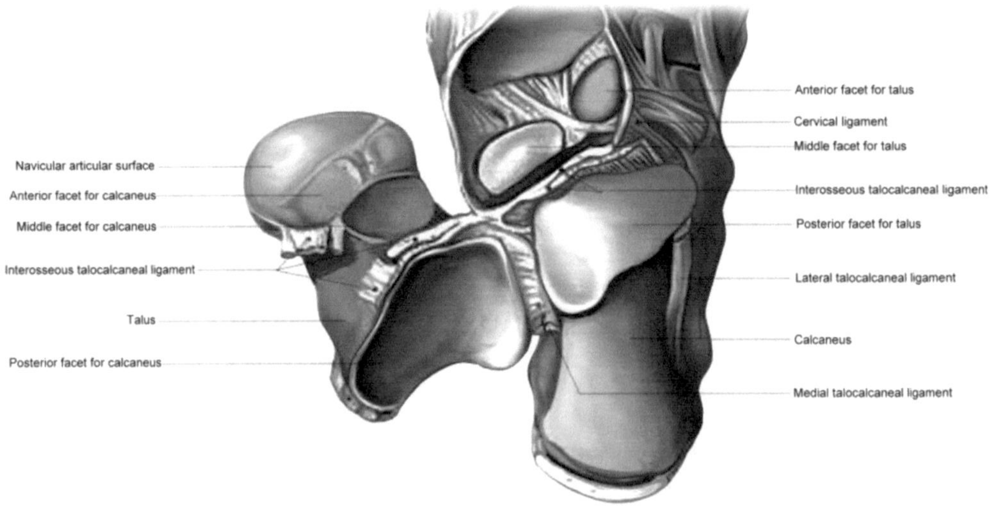

Figure 1. The subtalar joint

http://dx.doi.org/10.5772/55112

3. Indication and contraindication

The diagnostic indications of subtalar arthroscopy include persistent pain, swelling, catching, locking or instability resistant to conservative treatment. The therapeutic indications include chondromalacia, osteoarthritis, osteochondral lesions, synovitis, plica syndrome, loose body, ligament injury and posterior impingement syndrome of the hindfoot.

The absolute contraindications include localized infection, as well as severe degenerative joint disease or deformity. The relative contraindications include arthrofibrosis with severely narrow joint space, poorly vascularized extremity and neuropathic joint disease. Severe edema mentioned as a relative contraindication in previous literatures[8] has not been a contraindication yet since portals are not difficult to make by experienced arthroscopists even without obvious bony landmarks.

4. Surgical technique of subtalar arthroscopy

The instrument used for subtalar arthroscopy is similar to that used in ankle joint. Usually a 30° 2.7mm arthroscopy is used for subtalar joint. A 30° 1.9mm arthroscopy is used in some cases with tight joints and 4.0mm arthroscopy can be used in those with large joints. 2.9mm shaver and burr are routine instruments for subtalar arthroscopy. Small punch and probe should be also available. Other instruments such as small curette and microfracture device are optional. (Figure 2)

Supine position with elevation of pelvic region by a cushion and general or local anesthesia are usually used. The tourniquet is applied to the proximal thigh and inflated under pressure of 250mmHg to 350mmHg. Distraction belt is used in all patients. Bony distraction is seldom used except for small joints.

Initially the subtalar joint is distended by injection of normal saline in the subtalar joint using the anterolateral portal. Two anterolateral portals and two posterolateral portals are used for subtalar arthroscopy. The anterolateral (AL) portal is at 1cm distal and 2cm anterior to the fibular tip. The anterior anterolateral (AAL) portal is at 3cm anterior to the fibular tip. The posterolateral (PL) portal is at 0.5cm proximal to the fibular tip and just lateral to the Achilles tendon. The other portal is anterior posterolateral (APL) portal which is between the AL portal and the PL portal just behind peroneal tendons. After distending the joint the AL portal is firstly made for arthroscopic exploration with skin incision and subcutaneous separated bluntly. The AAL portal is then made for instrument placing. After exploring the joint from the AL portal arthroscopy is switched to the PL portal for further exploring the posterior part of the subtalar joint. Frey et al[3] reported that the best portal combination for access to the cartilaginous posterior facet of the subtalar joint involved placing the arthroscope through the AAL portal and the instrumentation through the PL portal. This allows directly visualization and instrumentation of nearly the entire surface of the posterior facet and involved contents. (Figure 3)

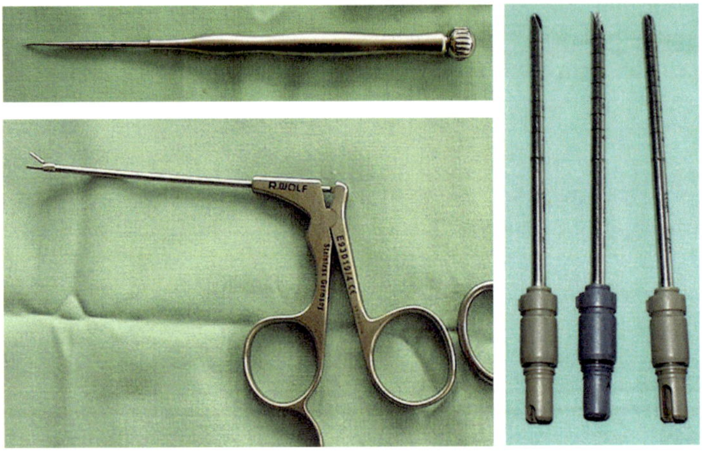

Figure 2. Instruments for subtalar arthroscopy (small probe, punch, shaver & burr)

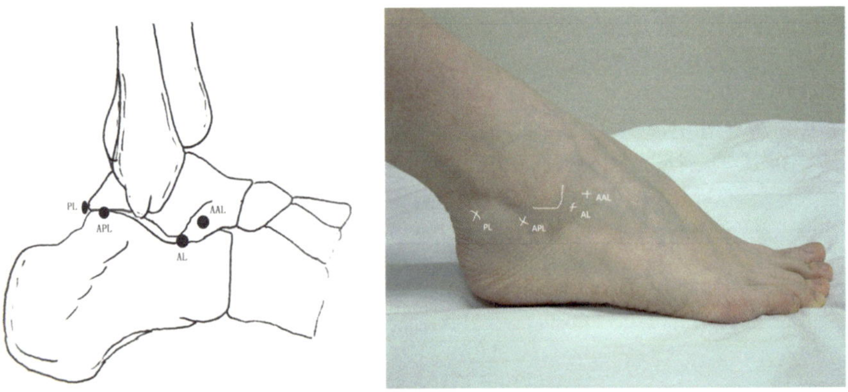

Figure 3. Portals for subtalar arthroscopy

The exploration starts from insertion of arthroscope through the AAL portal and placing probe through the AL and PL portals. The posterior subtalar joint is explored in the order of deep interosseous ligament, superficial interosseous ligament, anterolateral corner, lateral gutter and the central articulation. Arthroscope is then switched to the PL portal and the probe is placed through the AL and AAL portals. Exploration is done in the order of interosseous talocalcaneal ligament anteriorly, anterolateral corner, lateral gutter, posterior gutter, posteromedial gutter, posteromedial corner and the posterior aspect of the talocalcaneal joint. (Figure 4~Figure 5)

http://dx.doi.org/10.5772/55112

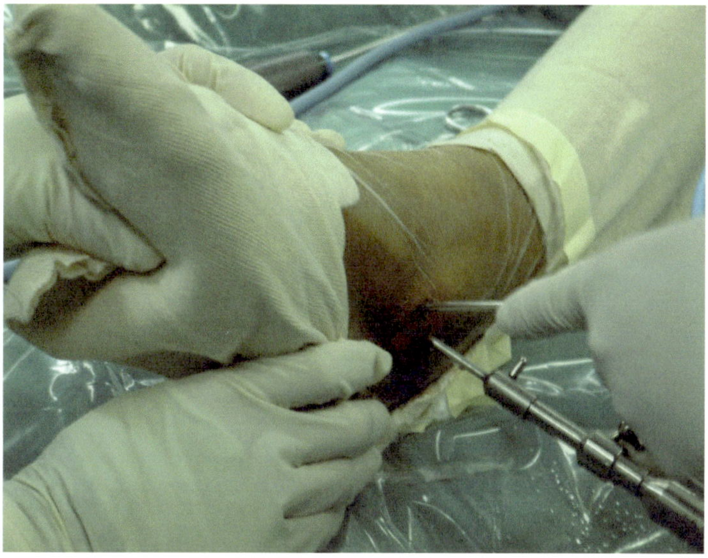

Figure 4. Insertion of arthroscopy

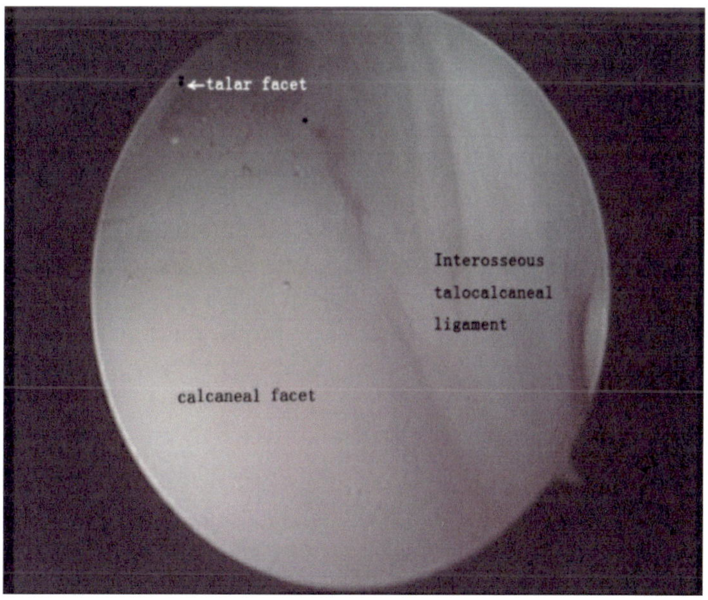

Figure 5. Subtalar joint under arthroscopy (View from the AL portal)

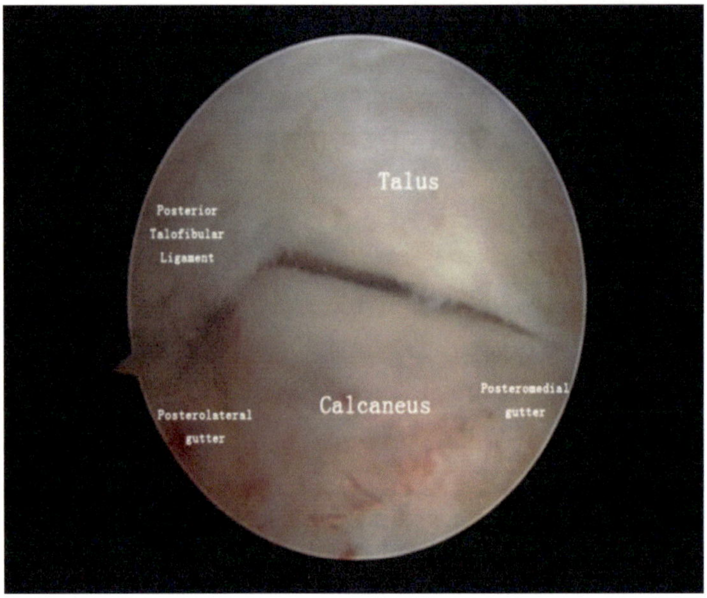

Figure 6. Subtalar joint under arthroscopy (View from the PL portal)

Therapeutic manipulation is done following exploration. Cartilage debridement, microfracture or loose body removal is performed for chondromalacia, osteoarthritis or osteochondral lesions. Synovectomy is performed for synovitis or plica syndrome. Os trigonum resection is done for posterior impingement syndrome of the hindfoot. The surgical technique refers to relative chapters on the knee and the ankle. The ligament reconstruction for subtalar instability (ITCL rupture) is described in detail below.

5. Surgical technique of Interosseous talocalcaneal ligament reconstruction

The ITCL is the main soft tissue stabilizer of the subtalar joint. Rupture of the ITCL can be associated with ankle sprains especially when combined with subtalar dislocation. Patients with chronic injury of the ITCL have symptoms of pain and swelling located in the tarsal sinus and instability of the hindfoot. Although relatively uncommon, and probably underreported in the literature, such problems were sometimes misdiagnosed as sinus tarsi syndrome. Now with an improved understanding of anatomy and function of the ITCL and the development of radiological diagnostic techniques, the differences between these two types of disease are apparent.

Physical examinations are critical for diagnosis of the ITCL injury. The anterior drawer test[9] of the subtalar joint was positive in patients with the ITCL injury when the affected foot was compared to the uninjured foot. We also designed calcaneal transverse slide test and calcaneal tilt test for diagnosis. The calcaneal transverse slide test is performed with one hand fixing the talus and the other hand pulling the calcaneus transversely to feel a slide between two bones.

http://dx.doi.org/10.5772/55112

The calcaneal tilt test is performed in the same way to feel inversion of the calcaneus "and opening up" on the lateral side of the subtalar joint.

The stress radiograph to measure the displacement of the calcaneus against the talus and subtalar tilt angle is more reliable[10,10,11]. However, the instrument used and standard for diagnosis differed among literatures. The ITCL can be clearly observed on MRI which is valuable for diagnosis and assessment in follow-up.

The surgical technique was designed in 2008[12]. The arthroscopy is performed with the patient in supine position and under general or spinal anaesthesia. The hip of affected side is lifted with internally rotation of the tibia. A thigh tourniquet was then inflated with pressure of 300mmHg. An AAL portal and an AL portal are established initially. The subtalar joint is then explored under arthroscopy. Rupture of ITCL and the remnant of the ligament can be observed. The calcaneal transverse slide test and the calcaneal tilt test are more obvious under arthroscopy. The articulation is explored under arthroscopy. Cartilage injury and synovitis can be treated simultaneously. The remnant of the ITCL is removed.

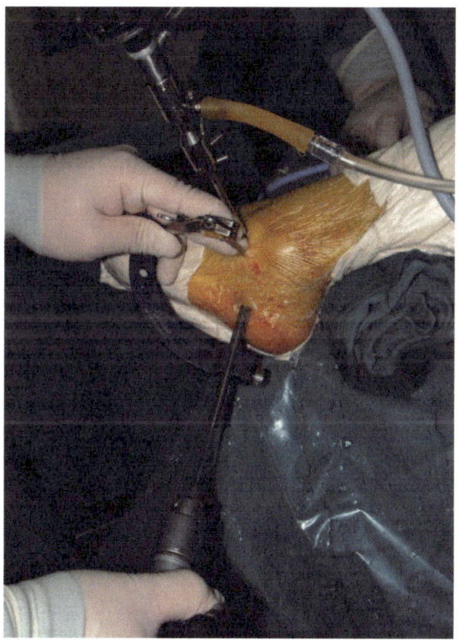

Figure 7. Making the calcaneal under arthroscopy

Before drilling the positions of bone tunnels are marked with radiofrequency. The anterolateral portal and the lower anteromedial portal are made in ankle for aiming of the outer exit of the bone tunnel of the talus. Two tunnels, 4.5 mm in diameter, are made in the talus and the calcaneus with the aimer (Figure 7 to Figure 10). The talar tunnel is located at the foot print of the ITCL medial to the anterior-lateral corner of the posterior facet and drilled toward the superomedial corner of the talar neck. The calcaneal tunnel is located at the remnant of the calcaneal root of the ITCL at a sulcus medial to the anterolateral corner of the posterior subtalar facet of the calcaneus and drilled toward the lateral side of calcaneus. A gracilis tendon is obtained from the ipsilateral knee. It is trimmed and sutured to double-bundle with 4mm to

4.5mm in diameter and about 10 cm in length. No.2 polyester sutures were placed at each end. This double-strand ligament is passed through two bone tunnels and fixed with two 4.5mm Bio-Corkscrew suture anchors (Arthrex) in the bone tunnels as interference screws under arthroscopy while the foot is held in a neutral position (Figure 11 and Figure 12). The negative instability exams are performed at the end of operation under arthroscopy and manually.

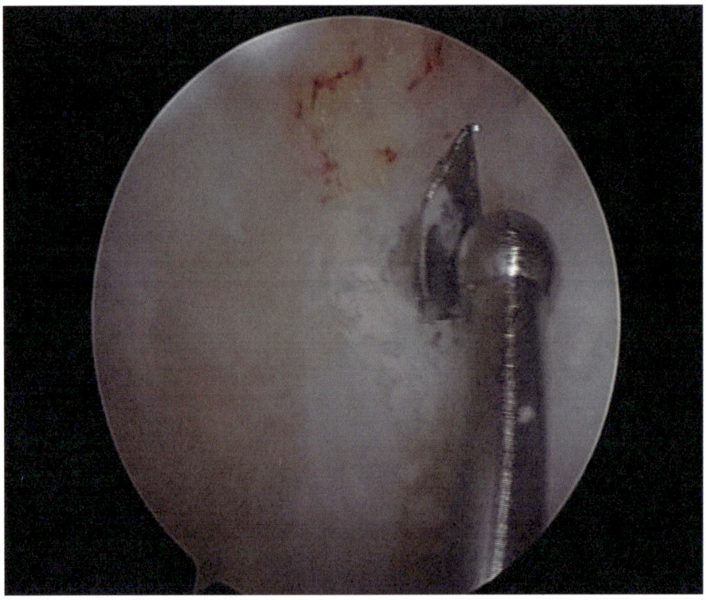

Figure 8. Making the calcaneal bone tunnel bone tunnel

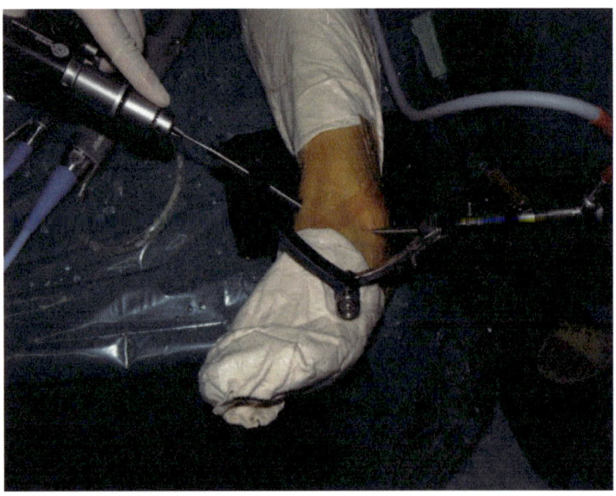

Figure 9. Making the talar bone tunnel under arthroscopy

http://dx.doi.org/10.5772/55112

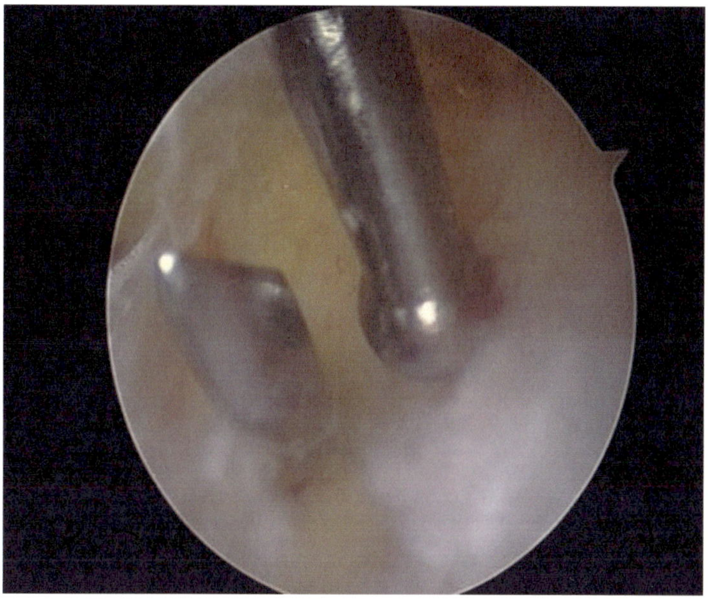

Figure 10. Making the talar bone tunnel

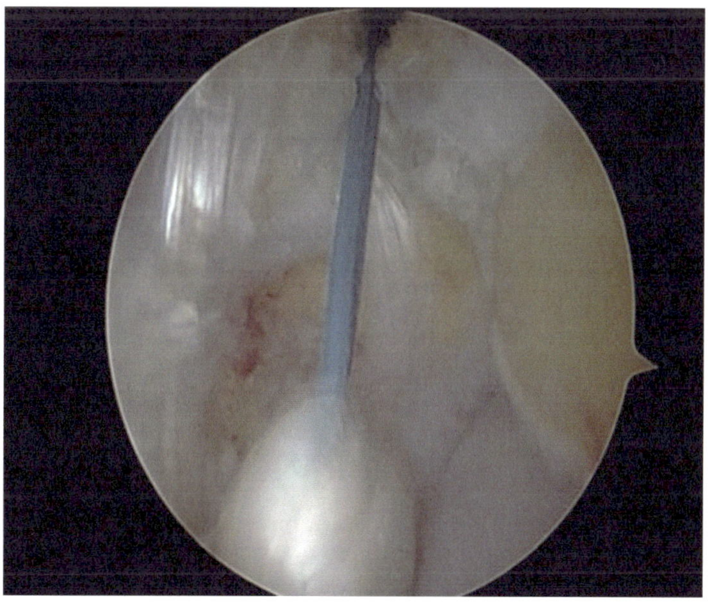

Figure 11. The gracilis tendon passing through bone tunnels

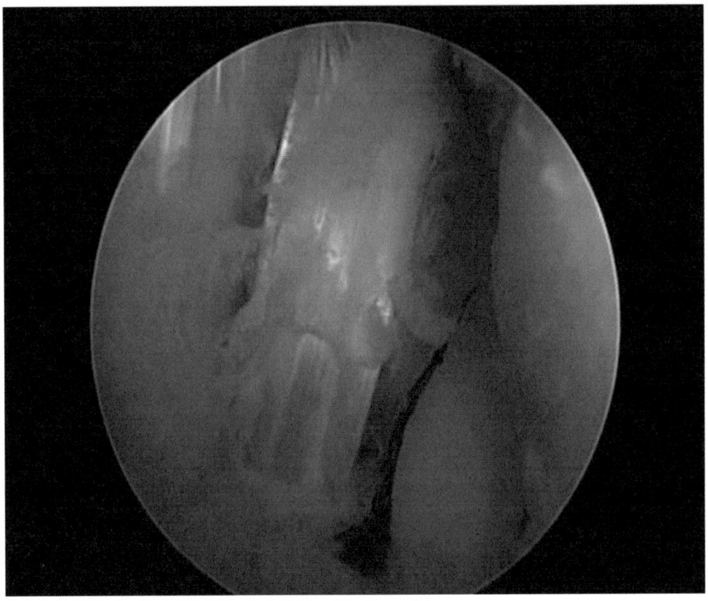

Figure 12. Reconstructed ITCL

6. Complication

The dorsal branches of superficial peroneal nerve, the third peroneus and the small saphenous vein located near the AAL portal can be injured when making the portal. The sural nerve and peroneal tendons can be injured when the APL portal is made. The Achilles tendon are probably injured when doing the PL portal. There is no severe complication for subtalar arthroscopy.

7. Postoperative rehabilitation

After subtalar arthroscopy the hindfoot is compressed with an elastic bandage or a cotton splint for two days. Then, half weight bearing and range of motion (ROM) exercise starts. Full weight bearing begins 2 weeks after surgery. The ROM exercise completes in four weeks. Patients return to daily life and sports 6 to 8 weeks after operation.

After the ITCL reconstruction the hindfoot is immobilized in a compressive cotton splint for 3 days. After removal of this dressing a hindfoot brace is applied with the foot in neutral position for 8 to 10 weeks. The ROM exercise is encouraged a week after surgery. Partial weight bearing begins 6 weeks after operation and full weight bearing is encouraged at 8 weeks. Patients return to normal ROM and walking 3 months after the operation and return to sports 6 to 9 months after the operation.

Author details

Jiao Chen, Hu Yuelin and Guo Qinwei
Institute of Sports Medicine, Peking University Third Hospital, China

References

[1] Kieser, C. W, & Jackson, R. W. SeverinNordentoft: The first arthroscopist". Arthroscopy (2001)., 17(5), 532-535.

[2] Parisien, J. S, & Vangsness, T. Arthroscopy of the subtalar joint- An experimental approach. Arthroscopy (1985)., 1(1), 53-57.

[3] Frey, C, Gasser, S, & Feder, K. Arthroscopy of the subtalar joint. Foot ankle int (1994)., 15(8), 424-428.

[4] Lundeen, R. O. Arthroscopic fusion of the ankle and subtalar joint.ClinPodiatr Med Surg (1994)., 11(3), 395-406.

[5] Sizer, P. S. jr., Phelps P, James R, Matthijs O. Diagnosis and management of the painful ankle/foot part 1:Clinical anatomy andpathomechanics. Pain Practice (2003)., 3(3), 238-262.

[6] Leardini, A, Stagni, R, & Conner, O. JJ. Mobility of thesubtalar joint in the intact ankle complex. J Biomech.(2001)., 34(6), 805-809.

[7] Astrom, M, & Arvidson, T. Alignment and joint motionin the normal foot. J Orthop Sports PhysTher. (1995)., 22(5), 216-222.

[8] Williams, M. M, & Ferkel, R. D. Subtalar arthroscopy: indications, technique and results. Arthroscopy (1998)., 14(4), 373-381.

[9] Kato T: The diagnosis and treatment of instability of the subtalar jointJ Bone Joint Surg Br.(1995)., 77(3), 400-406.

[10] Heilman, A. E, Braly, W. G, Bishop, J. O, et al. An anatomic study of subtalar instability. Foot ankle.(1990).

[11] Yamamoto, H, Yagishita, K, Ogiuchi, T, et al. Subtalar instability following lateral ligament injuries of the ankle. Injury.(1998)., 29(4), 265-268.

[12] Liu, C, Jiao, C, Hu, Y, et al. Interosseoustalocalcanealligament reconstructionwith hamstringautograftundersubtalar arthroscopy: case report. Foot Ankle Int (2011)., 32(11), 1089-1094.

Chapter 7

Shoulder Arthroscopy

Jeremy Rushbrook, Panayiotis Souroullas and
Neil Pennington

Additional information is available at the end of the chapter

http://dx.doi.org/10.5772/55005

1. Introduction

Shoulder arthroscopy has become increasingly popular as the modality of choice for interventional procedures in surgery. Results for treatment of instability and rotator cuff disease are comparable with open procedures, yet with much reduced morbidity. Some pathology (such as SLAP lesions), visualised and treated with much difficulty at an open procedure are more easily and successfully managed at arthroscopy. The greatest limitation to success is the difficulty in understanding the complex anatomy from the view of the arthroscope, and the principles of management for the common conditions. This chapter presents an overview of indications, technique, anatomy and treatment options to aid understanding.

2. History of shoulder arthroscopy

Shoulder arthroscopy was first performed in 1931 by the American Dr Michael Burman [1]. He developed techniques on cadavers of which many principles are still practiced today. These include joint distension using fluid or air, the use of traction for distraction and the importance of positioning. The Second World War slowed progression until Dr Masaki Watanabe began to modify arthroscopic equipment in the 1950's [2]. Development during subsequent decades produced smaller diameter arthroscopes, higher quality lenses, fibre-optic light sources and the charge coupled device (CCD) camera [3].

Clinical shoulder arthroscopy developed at a slower rate to that used in the knee, with the first application described by Andren and Lundbery in 1965 for the treatment of frozen shoulder [4]. Watanabe described the posterior portal in 1978 [5] and began to describe the anatomy of the shoulder as viewed through the arthroscope [6]. Conti shortly after described the anterior portal [7]. Shoulder arthroscopy soon became popular, especially in the treatment of dynamic glenohumeral joint and subacromial disorders. As techniques develop, arthroscopy has been used to perform acromiaclavicular joint stabilisations and excision, suprascapular nerve releases, bone block transfers and even latissimus dorsi transfers.

3. Indications

3.1. Diagnostic

Shoulder arthroscopy was initially introduced as a diagnostic procedure, and this remains an important part of its use. Both intra- and extra-articular shoulder structures are accessible with the arthroscope, which causes minimal tissue damage. Its use has led to the description of several pathological entities, such as the Superior Labrum Anterior Posterior (SLAP) lesion. The glenohumeral joint (GHJ), subacromial space, acromioclavicular joint (ACJ) and scapulothoracic articulation are all accessible. In addition, neurovascular structures such as the axillary nerve, suprascapular nerve, brachial plexus and axillary vessels are all within reach. Following examination under anaesthetic, a systematic diagnostic arthroscopy should be performed in all cases, before therapeutic intervention is initiated. This ensures all relevant pathology and abnormal anatomy is identified.

3.2. Therapeutic

3.2.1. Glenohumeral joint

Instability: Modes include a Bankart repair for anterior/inferior tears, capsular shrinkage / plication for atraumatic instability, as part of a Bankart repair or for internal impingement (Thrower's shoulder). In addition is the Latarjet procedure, now able to be performed arthroscopically, is found to be effective in 5 different scenarios: a. Instability with glenoid bone loss, b. Instability with humeral bone loss, c. combinations of glenoid and humeral bone loss, d. in cases of complex soft tissue injury (e.g. HAGL lesions) and finally e. as a revision procedure for failed Bankarts repairs [8].

- Cuff pathology: In cases of calcific tendinitis and rotator cuff tears
- Capsular pathology: Adhesive capsulitis intractable to NSAID's and physiotherapy.
- Biceps tendinopathies: SLAP lesions (proximal biceps-labrum complex lesions), tendon subluxation/dislocation, or biceps tendinopathy.
- Synovial disorders: Synovitis, Synovial chondromatosis and PVNS (Pigmented Villonodular Synovitis)
- Septic arthritis: Washout.
- Ganglia/Cysts: Decompression.
- Cartilage lesions (OA): Grafting.

3.2.2. Subacromial space

- Impingement
- Cuff pathology: Calcific tendinitis, rotator cuff tears.

3.2.3. Acromioclavicular joint

1. Instability
2. Dislocation
3. Degeneration

3.2.4. Suprascapular nerve

1. Entrapment: Nerve release

Scapulothoracic articulation

2. Snapping scapula: Bursitis, osteochondroma.

Muscle transfers

3. Large irreparable cuff tears: Arthroscopic Latissimus dorsi transfer.

4. Anaesthesia for shoulder arthroscopy

4.1. Examination under anaesthesia

A thorough history and clinical examination, supplemented by radiological examination leads to a correct diagnosis pre-operatively in the majority of cases. An examination under anaesthetic (EUA) will confirm such diagnoses, and can reveal valuable information that can occasionally lead to a change in the operative plan, such as unrecognised instability not detectable on clinical examination due to pain [9].

4.2. Passive range of movement

Passive range of movement is recorded in all planes, and attention must be paid to the point at which scapulothoracic movement commences. A comparison should always be made to the contralateral shoulder, particularly in the case of frozen shoulder. A goniometer can help quantify measurements.

4.3. Glenohumeral stability

Anterior and posterior translation should be performed and graded. Standing behind the patient, the scapula is stabilised with one hand whilst the other centralises the humeral head with an axial load, and then applies an anterior and posterior translation force. Grading is as follows:

- Grade 1 The humeral head can be translated to the glenoid rim
- Grade 2 The head subluxes over the glenoid rim but spontaneously reduces with release of force
- Grade 3 The head dislocated over the glenoid rim and remains dislocates after release

The test is performed in varying degrees of abduction and rotation when occult subluxation is suspected, and to allow the assessment of an engaging Hill-Sachs lesion [10].

5. Patient positioning [11]

Operating room setup and patient positioning are essential for the success of shoulder arthroscopy. Setup needs to allow sufficient space for the surgeon to move about freely, with one and possibly two assistants, the scrub nurse and all equipment to hand. A mayo table is usually positioned near the patients shoulder such that the surgeon is able to easily reach frequently needed equipment. The arthroscopy stack needs to be in a position that is easily viewed whilst operating, and the anaesthetist and anaesthetic equipment must not interfere with the surgeon. Blinds on windows should be drawn and room lights dimmed to facilitate viewing on the display. The patient is positioned either in the beach chair or lateral decubitus position, depending on surgeons preference. The patient is usually anaesthetised prior to positioning.

5.1. Lateral decubitus

The lateral decubitus is the traditional positioning for the shoulder arthroscopy, allowing excellent access and visualisation without the need of an assistant when balanced traction is applied. Following anaesthetic, the patient is positioned supine on the operating table to allow examination of both shoulders. An axillary roll can be placed on the unaffected side to protect the neurovascular bundle. The patient is then turned onto the contralateral side and held in position with pelvic supports. Pillows are placed between the legs and all bony prominences are padded. Special attention must be paid to the cervical spine to avoid excessive lateral flexion.

The arm can then either be placed into traction prior to preparing, or the entire arm can be prepped, and then placed into suspension, depending on surgeon preference and equipment availability. Traction load can be adjusted to provide distraction when required. The operating table is then tilted posteriorly by 30 degrees to position the glenoid parallel to the floor.

The lateral decubitus position allows gravity to work in favour of the surgeon, and makes the operation less physically demanding as the surgeons' elbows are kept by their side. Disadvantages include the need to lift and turn the patient, the possibility of excessive traction resulting in neurovascular injury, limited access to the anterior shoulder requiring repositioning if an open anterior approach is needed, and the tendency for suspension to place the arm in internal rotation.

http://dx.doi.org/10.5772/55005

5.2. Beach chair

The beach chair position has been adopted by many surgeons, and has been modified from the traditional position with the patient reclined at 45 degrees, to a more upright position. This allows easier orientation of the anatomy as it is in the more natural position of the patient, places the acromion parallel to the floor, and allows easier access to the posteroinferior shoulder.

The patient is anaesthetised supine and moved onto the operating table. The hips and knees are flexed as the patients back is raised to avoid the patient slipping down the table. A pillow can be placed below the knees and a footrest applied in addition. This seated position facilitates an interscalene block as either an adjunct to general anaesthetic, or as primary anaesthesia. Both shoulders are examined with the patient in this position. A variety of arm holder devices are available, with pneumatic devices becoming increasingly popular as they alleviate the need for an assistant to apply distraction to the arm.

Complications related to the beach chair position include transient hypotension and bradycardia particularly after interscalene block, known as the Bezold-Jarisch reflex, neurovascular injury particularly with pneumatic traction devices and intolerance to regional anaesthetic if used as the sole form of anaesthesia. Cardiac events and stroke are also more likely with the patient in a beach chair position.

6. Arthroscopic portals [12]

6.1. Introduction

An understanding of the normal anatomy of the glenohumeral joint is absolutely imperative in appreciating the position of several structures which are potentially at risk during an arthroscopic procedure. Equally important is spacial awareness of the subacromial space in positioning the arthroscopic portals depending on the indications as well as the desired outcome.

6.2. Positioning of portals

To the expert surgeon, portal entry is fairly simple and almost always intuitive. Positioning of the patient and choice of portal entry are essential in allowing for satisfactory view of the structures and joint, economy of movement aiming for minimum damage to soft tissues and neurovascular structures and finally in permitting the unhindered handling of instruments.

6.3. General technique

The commonest advice in approaching the joint for portal entry involves starting at the "soft spot" and aiming towards the coracoid. This is only slightly helpful as actual entry requires precision, and a deviation of even 3-5mm from the desired or intended position may render the operation technically difficult.

Marking the bony anatomical landmarks, which tend to be the most reliable in terms of a fixed location, greatly assisting in identifying the correct position for portal placement. Anteriorly, the coracoid process (CP), the acromioclavicular joint (ACJ) and the anterior border of the acromion are located and marked with a surgical site pen. Laterally, the lateral border of the acromion is palpated. More importantly, posteriorly and laterally lies the posterolateral corner of the acromion, a landmark that can be palpated even in obese patients. The scapula spine is also palpated and outlined on the patient. One may also choose to mark the biceps tendon in the bicipital groove, and the conjoint tendon. A bursal orientation line can be constructed with the posterior ACJ edge as the starting point, extending 4cm laterally and down the arm. This line marks the start of the subacromial bursa, proves the anterior nature of its position and can be particularly helpful in the placement of the lateral portal.

One must continuously remember that scope movement through the portal resembles movement through an hourglass with a pivot point (narrow point) at the portal level. The scope normally utilized is a 30-degree scope and alterations to the direction of the lens by means of rotation of the light source allow for an improved 3-dimensional perspective of the anatomy under assessment. Introduction of a probing needle is used as a confirmation tool prior to formation of a definitive portal in an attempt to optimize portal positioning and ensure adequate access to the structures under investigation.

Basic portals will be named A to E followed by F to K for the potentially more advanced ones.

6.4. Posterior Portal / Portal A: Glenohumeral and subacromial portal

Conventionally, surgeons describe entry for this portal at the "soft spot". This is traditionally located 2cm inferiorly and 1cm medially to the posterolateral acromial edge. A needle is advanced towards the coracoid and into the inferior apex of the triangle formed superiorly by the acromion, laterally by the humeral head and medially by the glenoid. As mentioned before, the needle acts as a directional guide pointing towards the joint. Occasionally, one may witness a hissing sound, which serves as a confirmation that the needle is within intra-articular space. A 5mm skin incision is then made and the arthroscope containing a blunt trocar is inserted into the joint. The contralateral hand of the surgeon is placed at the tip of the coracoid and the trocar is directed towards the middle finger of that hand, in an attempt to aid in the correct insertion. in the more technically challenging cases, the apex of the triangle, i.e. the joint line, can also be visualized by carefully riffling the scope tip over the posterior glenoid edge, before advancing it straight into the joint. Once the scope successfully enters the joint space, there is a feeling of "give".

The camera can then be inserted to confirm visualization of the following structures:

1. Anterior capsule, glenohumeral ligaments, rotator cuff intervals, superior 1/3 of subscapularis, intraarticular biceps tendon inferior recess of the labrum, glenoid and humeral surfaces, supraspinatus and infraspinatus muscles.

2. Internervous plane: plane between infraspinatus(suprascapular nerve) and teres minor (axillary nerve).

http://dx.doi.org/10.5772/55005

3. Structures at risk: Axillary nerve, posterior circumflex humeral vessels. The posterior deltoid fibres, as well as infraspinatus fibres may be traversed by way of this portal.

Even though this approach gives sufficient access to the glenohumeral space/joint, there is an obvious technical disadvantage in attempting to use the same portal for gaining adequate access to the subacromial space. Because the arthroscopic view via this portal is directed medially, the lateral insertion of the rotator cuff cannot be adequately visualized. Furthermore, because of the superior angle of the scope, it is more difficult to produce a "bird's eye" view of the rotator cuff thus not allowing for a good appreciation of potential rotator cuff lesions.

Consequently, the first portal is slightly modified to gain access to the subacromial space. Upon completion of the glenohumeral joint examination. The scope is reintroduced with the trochar but redirected towards the anterolateral corner of the acromion. A sweeping motion is also used to tidy up any adhesions prior to pushing fluid through to re-initiate joint distention. The camera is then reinserted and a bursoscopy is performed.

Structures seen using this approach include:

1. subacromial space, ACJ, bursal aspect of the rotator cuff, extra-articular biceps, coracoid and the coracoacromial ligament.
2. The posterior deltoid fibres are once again at risk.

A second posterior portal also becomes necessary owing to the aforementioned technical difficulties.

6.5. Portal B – Posteriolateral portal : Subacromial

This portal serves as an access point to the posterior labrum and posterior rotator cuff aspects. Entry point is traditionally found at 1cm antero-inferior to the posterolateral edge of the acromion.

This portal is often used in posterior Bankart lesion repairs, instrumented repairs and suture managements, and allows visualization of the above mentioned structures when advanced.

Once again, the posterior deltoid fibres may be traversed, and there is a risk of damage to infraspinatus particularly if the portal is used to instrument articular structures. The axillary nerve is now in close proximity lying only 4-5cm inferior to the portal entry point.

6.6. Portal C – Lateral subacromial portal

This constitutes the first portal in cases where the intended procedure includes subacromial decompression, adhesive capsulitis release, or repair of massive rotator cuff tear.

The entry point is located at the midpoint if the acromion, the location of which is once again confirmed by means of needle insertion. This location provides for good access to the subacromial space, as well as visualization, manipulation and repair of cuff tears.

Overall this portal is probably the most functional in terms of diagnostic and interventional procedures.

Structures best visualized include subacromial space, ACJ, bursal side of rotator cuff, suprascapular nerve, coraco-clavicular ligaments, extra-articular biceps, coracoid, coraco-acromial ligament, coraco-humeral ligament, rotator interval, extra-articular subscapularis and the conjoint tendon.

Structures at risk include posterior fibres of the deltoid as well as the axillary nerve.

6.7. Portal D – Superolateral portal

This portal is ideal in providing access to the biceps tendon and the subscapularis insertion, as well as the anterior labrum rim and neck. It is also known as the sub-bicipital portal and and its positioning is best achieved by advancing a spinal needle 1cm from antero-lateral edge of the acromion. Furthermore, it can be used for single or double row repairs of the anterior labrum (Casseiopia technique).

In cases of intact cuff, intra-articular access is achieved by traversing the coracohumeral ligament and the rotator interval where the ligament can be positively identified from its insertion on the coracoid.

Such approach provides for intra-articular access, but also access to the sub-coracoid space which is particularly useful in plexus exploration, subscapularis release, instrumentation of the supra-coracoid space in suprascapular nerve exposure.

Structures identified include supraspinatus, subscapularis, rotator interval, coracoid, sub-coracoid space and bursa, suprascapular nerve and intra-articular space via the rotator interval. Structures at risk of damage include anterolatral deltoid, rotator interval and biceps tendon.

6.8. Portal E – Anterior portal

Creation of this portal is an essential constituent in the diagnostic arthroscopy by allowing appropriate instrument access, thus providing for proper palpation and dynamic examination of the various shoulder structures.

The secret behind successful creation of this portal lies in the ability to visualise the biceps tendon and the rotator interval as seen through the posterior portal. To start off, a needle is inserted using the outside in technique, in an attempt to confirm the best portal position and to probe normal anatomy. The key anatomical landmark is located halfway along a line drawn from the acromion to the coracoid. It is essential to remain lateral to the coracoid in order to minimise the risk of damage to the neurovascular structures.

Following confirmation of the correct needle position via the intra-articular view, a skin incision is made with the blade advanced into the rotator interval using the needle as a guide, always being careful not to damage adjacent structures. Alternative instrument introductory methods include the use of a blunt trocar to penetrate the anterior capsule, the use of a cannulated portal or implementation of techniques which involve the use of a switching stick.

This portal is traditionally used in anterior instrumentation but also allows for an alternative view of the biceps anchor, anterior labrum and glenoid neck, as well as view of the subscapularis, infraspinatus, teres minor, posterior labrum and capsule.

Of note is that this portal transgresses the anterior deltoid fibres as well as the rotator interval thus putting these structures at risk. Medially, one needs to be aware of the brachial plexus and axillary vessels, inferolaterally the musculocutaneous nerve and finally the cephalic vein.

7. Anatomy of the shoulder as viewed through the arthroscope

7.1. Glenohumeral joint

Once intra-articular access has been obtained with the arthroscope, a systematic examination of the shoulder is performed. This usually begins with the gleno-humeral joint. Thorough knowledge of the anatomy and normal variants is essential both to recognise pathology, and to avoid repairing a normal variant, in the mistaken belief that it is a pathological lesion.

7.2. Capsule

The capsule can be considered a watertight structure that acts to restrain the joint but permit the great range of movement of the shoulder. The volume of the joint is determined by the capsule, and varies significantly from the small, restrictive volume in patients with adhesive capsulitis, to the capacious capsule in those with connective tissue disorders or multidirectional instability.

The capsule incorporates both the tendons of the rotator cuff as they approach their insertions, and the glenohumeral ligaments, which are seen as localised thickenings. The capsule is lined by synovium, and is therefore susceptible to inflammatory disorders, malignancy and tumour-like conditions.

7.3. Glenohumeral ligament

The superior glenohumeral ligament (SGHL) is seen in 40-94% of shoulder and tends to have the most consistent anatomy of the three anterior ligaments. It usually arises at the 12 o'clock position at the supra glenoid tubercle, but can also originate from the biceps anchor and labrum. It travels parallel to the biceps tendon to insert on the medial edge of the bicipital groove and the fovea capitus.

Laterally, the SGHL joins the coracohumeral ligament, contributes to and stabilises the biceps pulley and forms part of the rotator interval. Visibility of the ligament is improved by adducting the shoulder.

The middle glenohumeral ligament (MGHL) is present in 84-92% of shoulders, and has a more variable position than the SGHL, originating from the upper part of the glenoid, the labrum, or from the origination of the SGHL. It separates from the SGHL, where it is easily visible, runs diagonally downward and across the tendon of subscapularis to insert into the lesser tuberosity. The interval between the two ligaments forms the entrance to the subscapular bursa through the foramen of Weitbrecht. This space can be utilised arthroscopically to perform subscapularis release and to approach the brachial plexus and subscapular nerves.

The appearance of the MGHL is subject to common variations, appearing either as a cord-like structure, absent or thin ligament, or a part of a Buford complex which comprises a cord like MGHL arising from the superior labrum with an absent anterior superior labrum. The variation in morphology may play a role in the aetiology of SLAP tears by contributing to the stress on the biceps anchor.

Attention should always be payed to the humeral insertion to avoid missing a humeral avulsion of the glenohumeral ligaments (HAGL). Below the MGHL is the inferior subscapular recess which corresponds to the subcoracoid foramen of Rouviere.

The inferior glenohumeral ligament (IGHL) is present in 75-93% of shoulders and comprises an anterior band (IGHLa) which originates from the glenoid between the 2 and 5 o'clock position, and a posterior band (IGHLp) which originates from the 7 to 9 o'clock position. These converge to form a sling which inserts on the humerus in the 4 to 8 o'clock position. The intervening capsular tissue between the two bands represents the axillary pouch. Due to its arrangement, the IGHL forms the main static stabiliser of the GHJ in abduction, and therefore should be carefully visualised.

7.4. Labrum

This ring of fibrous tissue forms a circumferential lip around the glenoid and provides a static role in glenohumeral stability by deepening the socket by up to 50%. It also provides an origin for the glenohumeral ligaments and biceps anchor. Anatomical variations are most commonly seen in the anterosuperior segment, with a sub-labral foramen being reported in 12-19% of shoulders.

These can be easily confused with a traumatic anterior labral injury (Bankart lesion) but need to be differentiated as the unwarranted repair can lead to a poor outcome. More inferiorly the labrum attaches to the glenoid in a consistent manner with good fixation to bone.

7.5. Rotator interval

The rotator interval (RI) is located in the anterior shoulder and is implicated in various pathologies, particularly with regard to instability and stiffness. It is triangular in shape with its base at the coracoid process, its apex at the intertubercular groove, its inferior margin the superior border of the subscapularis tendon, and its superior margin the inferior border of the supraspinatus tendon.

The contents of the (RI) are the SGHL, biceps tendon, the coracohumeral ligament (CHL), and the glenohumeral joint capsule. The function of the RI and its components is to restrict inferior and posterior translation of the humeral head via the SGHL and CHL as well as limiting external rotation.

http://dx.doi.org/10.5772/55005

Its lateral components maintain the stability of the biceps tendon. The RI also maintains negative intra-articular pressure. Lesions of the RI have been classified into two types.

Type I lesions are those leading to a contracture of the RI e.g. adhesive capsulitis, and type II lesions lead to laxity.

7.6. Coracohumeral ligament

This trapezoid structure is located in the rotator interval. It originates from an extra-articular location via two roots; a ventral root arising from the anterior part of the dorsolateral coracoid, and a dorsal root from the base of the coracoid. Both roots lie beneath the CA ligament, after which the CHL takes a course parallel to the long head of biceps tendon and through the RI. Its insertion laterally is subject to variation, its most common position being into the RI itself. Occasionally the CHL inserts into the supraspinatus tendon, subscapularis tendon, or both.

The CHL is thought to represent a remnant of a redundant pectoralis minor ligament, but is thought to contribute to limiting external rotation with the arm in abduction, as well as providing resistance to inferior translation of the humeral head. It is also thought to be the primary structure affected by adhesive capsulitis and therefore surgical release should address this.

7.7. Biceps tendon

The long head of biceps tendon (LHBT) is an intra-articular structure but remains extra-synovial. It is enveloped in a synovial sheath which terminates at the distal end of the bicipital groove in a blind pouch. The importance of the LHBT is in providing a useful anatomical landmark for orientation, but also is a source of of pathology and symptoms.

The biceps tendon comprises three sections: the biceps anchor, the intra-articular tendinous portion, and the pulley system.

The biceps anchor originated from the supraglenoid tubercle and the glenoid labrum, and is the site of the Superior Labral Anterior Posterior lesion (SLAP), commonly seen in overhead throwing athletes and after traction injuries. The anchor is best visualised with the arm placed in abduction and external rotation using the Peel back test.

From its origin, the LHBT passes obliquely along the RI before exiting through the pulley system, this intra-articular section being on average 100mm in length. It is stabilised at is exits the shoulder via the pulley system prior to entering the bicipital groove. The pulley has four components, comprising the subscapularis tendon forming the floor, the CHL which forms the roof and lateral wall along with a tendinous slip of the supraspinatus tendon, and the SGHL forming the medial sling.

The supraspinatus and subscapularis tendons should be carefully assessed in cases of biceps tendon instability, which can be dynamically tested by performing internal and external rotational movements. Dislocation is manifested by the tendon moving completely out of its groove.

7.8. Rotator cuff

The rotator cuff tendons lie beneath the deltoid and are vital in enabling movement and providing stability to the shoulder joint. The cuff comprises four muscles - supraspinatus, infraspinatus, subscapularis and teres minor.

Subscapularis is the largest of the rotator cuff muscles, originating from the upper 2/3 of the anterior surface of the scapula, and condensing laterally to pass beneath the coracoid. The upper 2/3 in mostly tendinous, whilst the lower third remains muscular to its attachment point on the lesser tubercle adjacent to the biceps tendon. Internal rotation improves visibility of the insertion, which should be inspected carefully for evidence of a tear in the presence of an anterior pulley rupture, which can be classified as follows:

- **i.** Partial lesion only involving the upper 1/3 of subscapularis
- **ii.** Complete lesion of the upper 1/3
- **iii.** Complete lesion of the upper 2/3
- **iv.** Complete lesion of the tendon but the head remains centred and Goutallier ≤3
- **v.** Complete lesion with eccentric head position, coracoid impingement and Goutallier ≥4 (Goutallier grades refer to fatty degeneration of the muscle belly)

The supraspinatus muscle arises from the supraspinatus fossa via two muscle bellies to insert onto the greater tuberosity. The anterior fusiform belly gives rise to a central tendon which migrates anteriorly and forms an external extra-muscular tendon comprising 40% of the overall width of the tendon. The posterior 60% arises from a unipennate muscle belly. The difference in sizes results in 2.88 times greater stress in the anterior portion, which may be the cause for this being a common site of tearing.

The supraspinatus tendon is divided into four structurally independent subunits:

Tendon proper: extends from the musculotendinous junction to 2cm medial to the greater tuberosity. The collagen fibres in this region are parallel.

Rotator cable: a densely packed band of unidirectional collagen fibres extending from the CHL anteriorly to the inferior border of infraspinatus posteriorly which surrounds the thinner crescent, acting as a stress shield and causing maintenance of function even when there is a tear of the rotator crescent.

Fibrocartilage attachment: extends from the tendon proper to the greater tuberosity.

Capsule: composed of thin collagen sheets with a uniform fibre alignment.

Supraspinatus inserts into the superior and middle facets of the greater tuberosity, extending 1mm from the articular surface to a distance approximately 16mm lateral to it. This large footprint forms the basis of the double row technique of rotator cuff repair.

The thick, triangular, multipennate infraspinatus arise from the infraspinous fossa, converging into a tendon that passes across the posterior aspect of the glenohumeral joint. The tendon overlaps and joins the posterior border of the supraspinatus tendon, inserting into a trapezoidal footprint on the middle facet of the greater tuberosity with average dimensions of 29 ° ¡ 19mm, providing a large base for tendon to bone healing. The footprint narrows inferiorly, and the gap thus created forms the bare area.

Teres minor originates from the dorsal surface of the lateral border of the scapula and the fascia of infraspinatus. As it passes laterally, posterior to the shoulder joint, it forms its tendon which comprises part of the capsule and inserts onto the inferior facet of the greater tuberosity. The inferior border of the teres minor tendon forms the superior border of the quadrilateral space which transmits the posterior circumflex humeral artery and axillary nerve.

7.9. Glenoid

The glenoid has three components: bone, articular cartilage and the labrum. It is shaped like an inverted comma with a broader inferior portion, and a thinner superior tail. The average vertical dimension is 35mm and horizantal dimension is 25mm. 75% of glenoids are retroverted with regard to the plane of the scapular, with 15° superior tilt. The glenoid fossa is covered by hyaline cartilage, which is thicker at the periphery than the centre in order to deepen the concavity. 50% of the depth of the glenoid is due to the bony structure, the remaining 50% is formed by the labrum. The glenoid should be inspected in its entirety, to include the labrum.

7.10. Humeral head

The humeral head forms 1/3 of a true sphere, with the articular surface orientated 25-35° retrovertely and 130° superiorly. The anterior border is limited by the lesser tuberosity and the lateral border by the greater tuberosity. Between the two lies the inter-tubercular groove.

A bare area exists on the posterolateral humeral head adjacent to the infraspinatus tendon which can be confused with a Hills-Sachs lesion. Visualisation of the humeral head requires it to be rotated, abducted and adducted to ensure an adequate inspection. Stability can be assessed by performing translational movements.

7.11. Subacromial space / Subacromial bursa

The subacromial bursa lies between the anterior rotator cuff and the acromion and is a synovial-lined sac that acts to reduce friction and improve gliding between the rotator cuff and coraco-acromial arch.

The bursa lies in the anterior half of the subacromial space and access is best obtained by directing the scope anteriolaterally to the corner of the acromion. Bursectomy is often required to improve visualisation of the rotator cuff, which is inspected for tears, their size, shape, tendon involvement and the quality of the tendon involved.

7.12. Coracoacromial Ligament (CAL)

This strong triangular ligament forms the anterior part of the coracoacromial arch. It is separated from the rotator cuff by the subacromial bursa and is strongly associated in impingement syndrome.

It originates from a large area on the lateral aspect of the coracoid and narrows to insert on the anteromedial and anteroinferior surfaces of the acromion. Often distinct bands can be seen anterolateral and posteromedially. It is especially important to fully visualise the anterolateral band as spurs occur and cause impingement.

7.13. Coracoid

The coracoid is found at the base of the neck of the glenoid and projects anteriorly before hooking anterolaterally and flattening, providing the site of attachment of several tendons and ligaments.

Superiorly are the coracoclavicular ligaments (conoid and trapezoid), inferiorly lies the conjoint tendon, laterally the CHL and CAL, and inferomedially the pectoralis minor tendon. Inferomedial to the coracoid lie the neurovascular structures of the plexus and axillary vessels. Passing directly beneath the coracoid is the tendon of subscapularis. The coracoid has been described as the lighthouse of the shoulder, and helps to orientate the surgeon.

7.14. Acromion

The acromion forms from three ossification centres, which usually fuse by the age of 25. Failure of any of these centres leads to an os acromiale, which is an incidental finding in 8%. The acromion is the insertion point of the coracoacromial ligament and forms an articulation with the clavicle. The shape of the acromion is though to predispose to impingement syndrome and rotator cuff pathology, with three types described by Bigliani:

- **i.** Flat
- **ii.** Curved
- **iii.** Hooked

Type III are thought to be associated in the aetiology of rotator cuff tears.

7.15. Acromioclavicular joint

The acromioclavicular joint (ACJ) is a diarthrodial joint with the articular surfaces separated by an intra-articular disc. The joint is usually orientated superolateral to inferomedial. The lateral end of the clavicle is convex and articulates with the concave acromion. The joint is covered by a thick capsule, especially on its anterior, medial and superior surfaces and identifying its location is facilitated by applying pressure to the clavicle and observing movement of the joint.

http://dx.doi.org/10.5772/55005

8. Common procedures

8.1. Arthroscopic subacromial decompression

Arthroscopic subacromial decompression (ASD) is one of the most commonly performed operations of the shoulder. The arthroscopic technique bares little resemblance to the original open acromioplasty described by Neer. The indications for ASD are controversial. There are many causes for an impingement syndrome in the shoulder, and few are relieved by ASD. The aim of ASD is to convert a pathological coracoacromial arch into a physiological one. Patients with primary extrinsic impingement syndrome of the anterior acromion, coracoacromial arch and acromioclavicular joint on the underlying biceps tendon and rotator cuff, and those with chronic secondary impingement due to tendinous rotator cuff degeneration resulting in the formation of subacromial osteophyte formation are the most responsive to ASD.

ASD should be considered only after failure of conservative management. This involves the use of non-steroidal anti-inflammatories, physiotherapy for scapular, rotator cuff and range of movement exercises, and activity modification. Those with normal bony anatomy usually respond well. Relative contraindications to ASD include patients with massive rotator cuff tear and significant underlying glenohumeral arthritis likely to require arthroplasty. Dispute remains as whether or not to perform ASD during rotator cuff repair, with good evidence for both sides of the argument, and therefore most surgeons decompress where there is preoperative clinical or arthroscopic evidence of impingement.

The acromion and its underside can be preoperatively visualised radiographically with Neer's supraspinatus view. Bigliani described three distinct anatomical shapes: type 1 - flat (divergent), type 2 - curved (congruent), and type 3 - hooked (stenotic). The hooked acromion described as type 3 is more likely to cause an impingement and is suitable for ASD.

The arthroscopic technique for subacromial decompression was first described by Johnson in 1986. In contrast to the open procedure, there is no requirement to remove full thickness bone from the anterior acromion which therefore spares detachment of the deltoid fascial attachment or resection of the coracoacromial ligament. The results of ASD are therefore superior to open acromioplasty. The aim of surgery is to create a type 1 or 2 acromion, both of which are physiological in their shape, and likely to relieve the impingement syndrome. This must be performed without damaging the coracoacromial arch which can lead to destabilisation of the glenohumeral joint and anterior subluxation of the head. This only rarely occurs in ASD, though was more common with an open acromioplasty due to the reforming of the coracoacromial ligament after partial resection. The ACJ can also contribute to pain, particularly with distal clavical or medial acromion osteophyte formation and can lead to persistent pain postoperatively if neglected.

ASD is performed following a full diagnostic arthroscopy. Most surgeons examine the glenohumeral joint before repositioning in the subacromial space with a posterior portal. Instruments are usually then introduced through the lateral portal. The soft tissue on the underside of the acromion is firstly debrided with cautery ablation or a shaver. Care must be taken to remain on the underside of bone, and not migrate laterally into the fibres of deltoid, which can be highly vascular. A burr is introduced to start debridement at the anterolateral corner of the acromion, before progressing medially and posteriorly, to include the ACJ and distal clavicle if required. The diameter of the burr is a guide as to how much bone has been resected. Care must be taken not to remove full thickness bone anteriorly as this will lead to detachment of deltoid. The acromion should be resected to a smooth surface with an even taper.

The most common complications associated with ASD include inadequate or uneven resection leading to persistence of symptoms, injury to deltoid or rotator cuff, and haemorrhage. Post operatively there needs be no restriction on passive range of movement. Pendulum exercises can be started immediately, with physiotherapy continuing the preoperative exercises. Return to light duty is usually within 1 to 2 weeks, but heavy labour should be delayed for 6 to 12 weeks.

8.2. Excision lateral end of clavicle

The acromioclavicular joint (ACJ) is exposed to substantial forces during arm loading, and is therefore susceptible to degeneration. The ACJ is a diarthrodial joint with hyaline cartilage articulations partly separated by a fibrocartilage disc. It however degenerates to a fibrocartilaginous joint by the age of 40. Stability of the ACJ joint is achieved by a combination of the dynamic constraints of the deltoid and trapezius crossing the joint, and the static acromioclavicular and coracoclavicular ligaments. Degeneration of the ACJ is secondary to either degeneration or instability. Weightlifters are a group of individuals susceptible to early degeneration due to a stress reaction in the distal clavicle, known as distal clavicular osteolysis.

Presentation can be acutely, following an injury resulting in instability and consequent pain and mechanical symptons, or more chronically due to the insidious degeneration and gradual loss of function with arthritis. Mild to moderate symptoms can be treated conservatively initially, with activity modulation, and corticosteroid injection. Injection of local anaesthetic can be useful as a diagnostic procedure to confirm diagnosis. When symptoms do not resolve, and impede on a patients lifestyle, excision of the lateral clavicle should be considered. Relative contraindications include cystic disease within the distal clavicle, and instability that may be more suitable to reconstruction.

Routine diagnostic arthroscopy should always initiate the procedure though a posterior portal. If subacromial decompression is anticipated a lateral portal is used to provide access for instrumentation. Bursectomy is required to visualise the ACJ, and may be assisted by the use of a needle placed into the joint or by manual displacement. Cautery is then used to strip the inferior joint capsule from the joint. An accessory anterior portal is often useful to provide access to the joint and will allow exposure of the distal clavicle. Care must be taken to expose the superioanterior and posterior corners of the joint whilst preserving the superior acromioclavicular ligament to avoid iatrogenic instability. Once exposure is completed, resection is performed with the use of a burr. 8-10 mm of resection usually relieves impingement whilst preserving the medial coracoclavicular ligaments. Resection can be estimated by the placement of an instrument of known diameter.

Postoperatively the shoulder only requires immobilisation for comfort, and range of movement can be initiated without delay. Normal activities can be resumed within 6 weeks, although heavy lifting should be delayed for at least 12 weeks to avoid stretching the weakened acromioclavicular ligaments.

9. The future of shoulder arthroscopy

The future of arthroscopic shoulder surgery is already beginning to flourish through advances in both the biological as well as its technological sectors. Tissue engineering is already being implemented in cartilage reconstructive/reparative surgery. Muscle and tendon engineering has become possible with numerous studies under way to explore the potential.

Recent advances in micro-electronics technology has resulted in the development of needle arthroscopes, approaching the size of an 18 gauge needle, allowing some of the procedures to be performed under local anaesthetic, sometimes in the clinic setting.

Most current research is looking at nanobot injection into the joint. Their function relies on manipulation of molecules of ethylene monomer, directing them towards areas where wear and tear has manifested itself. This results in a polymerisation reaction locally, allowing high density molecules to form.

10. Summary

Shoulder arthroscopy has not only provided us with another extremely significant surgical tool used in both diagnosis and treatment of shoulder conditions, but also an improved well rounded understanding of shoulder anatomy, and mechanics of different diseases which were previously misdiagnosed or undiagnosed altogether e.g. SLAP lesions.

The fact that this technique requires the ability to think as well as the manual dexterity to operate in a three dimensional perspective, always appreciating surrounding anatomy, depth and economy of movement, are all constituents of a rather steep but rapidly evolving learning curve.

Author details

Jeremy Rushbrook*, Panayiotis Souroullas and Neil Pennington

York Hospital Foundation Trust, UK

References

[1] Burman, M. Arthroscopy pr the direct visualisation of joint: An experimental cadaver study. J Bone Joint Surg, (1931). , 669-695.

[2] Watanabe, M, Takeda, S, & Ikeuchi, H. Atlas of Arthroscopy(1957). Tokyo: Igakin-Shoin.

[3] Johnson, L. Arthroscopy of the shoulder. Orthop Clin North Am, (1980). , 197-204.

[4] Andren, L, & Lundberg, B. Treatment of rigid shoulders by joint distension during arthroscopy. Acta Orthop Scand, (1965). , 45-53.

[5] Watanabe, M, Takeda, S, & Ikeuchi, H. Atlas of Arthroscopy(1978). New York: Igaku-Shoin.

[6] Watanabe, M. Arthroscopy: the present state. Orthop Clin North Am, (1979). , 505-522.

[7] Conti, V. Arthroscopy in rehabilitation. Orthop Clin North Am, (1979). , 709-711.

[8] Lafosse, L, & Boyle, S. Arthroscopic Latarjet procedure. J Shoulder Elbow Surg, (2010). , 2-12.

[9] Silliman, J, & Hawkins, R. Classification and physical diagnosis of instability of the shoulder. Clin Orthop Relat Res., (1993). , 7-19.

[10] Fitzpatrick, M, et al. The anatomy, pathology, and definitive treatment of rotator interval lesions: current concepts. Arthoscopy, (2003). Supplement 1): , 70-79.

[11] Abrams, J, & Bell, R. Arthroscopic rotator cuff surgery(2008). New York: Springer.

[12] Boyle, S, et al. Shoulder arthroscopy, anatomy and variants. Orthopaedics and Trauma, (2009). , 291-296.